WOUND MANAGEMENT IN S

A practical guide for veterinary nu

C000004299

For Elsevier:

Commissioning Editor: Mary Seager
Development Editor: Rita Demetriou-Swanwick
Project Manager: Joannah Duncan
Designer: Andy Chapman
Illustrator: Samantha Elmhurst

WOUND MANAGEMENT IN SMALL ANIMALS

A practical guide for veterinary nurses and technicians

Louise O'Dwyer BSc (Hons) VN Dip AVN (Surgical)

Head Veterinary Nurse, Pet Medics Veterinary Centre, Manchester, UK

Bruce Tatton BVSc CertSAS MRCVS

Veterinary Surgeon, Pet Medics Veterinary Centre, Manchester, UK

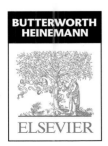

BUTTERWORTH HEINEMANN

ELSEVIER

Edinburgh London New York Oxford Philadelphia St Louis Sydney Toronto 2007

BUTTERWORTH
HEINEMANN
ELSEVIER

First published 2007

ISBN 0 7506 8831 9
ISBN-13 978 0 7506 8831 4

British Library Cataloguing in Publication Data
A catalogue record for this book is available from the British Library

Library of Congress Cataloging in Publication Data
A catalog record for this book is available from the Library of Congress

Knowledge and best practice in this field are constantly changing. As new research and experience broaden our knowledge, changes in practice, treatment and drug therapy may become necessary or appropriate. Readers are advised to check the most current information provided (i) on procedures featured or (ii) by the manufacturer of each product to be administered, to verify the recommended dose or formula, the method and duration of administration, and contraindications. It is the responsibility of the practitioner, relying on their own experience and knowledge of the patient, to make diagnoses, to determine dosages and the best treatment for each individual patient, and to take all appropriate safety precautions.
To the fullest extent of the law, neither the publisher nor the author assumes any liability for any injury and/or damage.

The Publisher

Printed in China

Contents

Acknowledgements

I am indebted to Paul Aldridge MRCVS for his many hours proofreading chapters, without which I am sure this book would never have come to fruition. Thanks additionally to Bruce Tatton MRCVS for his chapters on skin flaps and grafts and to Davina Anderson for her help and comments on Chapters 2 and 4.

Many thanks to Charlotte Bayes VN for the original line drawings for Chapters 6, 9 and 10.

This book hopefully provides the veterinary nurse with the basics for wound management, enabling a more knowledge based approach when faced with their next open wound which requires dressing and giving owners more information regarding the wound healing process.

My love goes to my mum for her many hours dog sitting.

Louise O'Dwyer
BSc (Hons) Dip AVN (Surgical) VN

Chapter 1

Introduction to wound management

Louise O'Dwyer

Veterinary nurses perform a vital and essential role within the operation of a practice. Veterinary nurses are now frequently involved in the establishment and running of their own clinics and consultations. These consultations frequently involve the assessment and treatment of patients following road traffic accidents, dog fights, etc. which often result in the patient sustaining a wound which will require treatment. The nurse may play an important role in the initial triage assessment and treatment of such wounds, followed by the evaluation of the wound with regard to closure options, dressings, etc. Such treatments may last for several weeks, meaning the veterinary nurse may be responsible for the selection of suitable dressings through the various stages of the healing process. This means a thorough and practical understanding of the dressings available is essential for the appropriate treatment of the patients.

Wound management has evolved radically over the years: early commentators recommended the use of olive oil dregs, lupine extract and good wine. As early as 200 BC writers were acknowledging the fact that infected wounds would not heal without the removal of infected tissue.

Evidence has been found throughout the centuries that various poultices were in use for the treatment of wounds on animals; these included warm ox urine and lanolin. Even these early treatments realised the importance of the cleansing of wounds, with warm wine being frequently recommended.

Lister and Pasteur were amongst the early scientists who realised the importance of antisepsis and sterility in surgical outcomes.

Wound dressings have evolved radically from these early times, but it is the continuous research by drug companies that produces the most effective dressings available for wound management that we see marketed today.

Successful wound management requires accurate assessment and planning in order to ensure a good outcome; part of this planning involves knowing and anticipating which dressing is most suitable.

No two wounds are the same and hence no single dressing is appropriate in all situations. This book aims to simplify the confusing array of wound dressings currently on the market, enabling the veterinary nurse to select the dressing which they feel is most appropriate for a particular wound to give the best possible outcome.

The priorities for wound management alter during the different phases of wound healing; therefore it is important to understand the ways in which the various dressings enhance the healing process so that the correct dressing can be selected.

Open wound management is at its most effective when the treatment supports and complements the natural healing process, and this is what we aim to do by applying the principles of moist wound healing.

We dress wounds for several different reasons:

- Protection from further trauma
- Protection from the patient
- Protection from contamination
- Provision of analgesia.

For these reasons dressings need to be hardwearing, waterproof, bacteria proof, absorbent, and have active cleansing properties.

The principles of surgical asepsis also need to be taken into consideration when looking at wound management; this is a particularly important aspect as post-operative wound infections are a common and serious complication of surgery, with the effects ranging from minor infections which may be quickly and easily resolved, to serious life-threatening illness which may be difficult and expensive to treat.

All aspects of the surgical technique need to be considered, from hair removal through to the theatre environment and preparation of the surgical team.

Indian history has references going back 3000 years in the Caraka Samhita, and 2500 years in the Shusrata Samhita, to the use of sutures in the closure of wounds. These records detail the use of early sutures in tonsillectomy, caesarean sections, amputations and rhinoplasty. During these early times the sutures were made from flax, hemp, bark fibre or hair. The jaws of large black ants were used to bite the wound edges together, so the powerful jaws acted as staples or clips.

Modern suture materials have greatly evolved to make specific material for use in different organs. Each suture has different properties making them particularly suitable for use in a particular structure, in terms of tensile strength, knot security, action of absorption. These factors all make the selection of the most appropriate suture material highly important and this is an area in which the veterinary nurse's knowledge of the particular properties of such sutures can play an important role when assisting the veterinary surgeon. This knowledge also helps the veterinary nurse when performing their own Schedule 3 procedures.

Hopefully by the end of this book the nurse will have gained the knowledge and confidence to go out and see these cases in action and gain satisfaction from seeing positive results in wound healing for all their hard work.

Further reading

Clewlow J 2003 A review of the history of veterinary wound management. Online. Available: www.worldwidewounds.com

Shales C J 2004 Principles of surgery: surgical asepsis. UK Vet 9(2): 20-30

Chapter 2
Wound assessment and management
Louise O'Dwyer

WOUND CLASSIFICATION

The following parameters can be used to classify wounds:

- Aetiology
- Nature and extent of the skin deficit
- Degree of bacterial contamination
- Extent of the trauma to the surrounding tissues.

TYPES OF WOUNDS

ABRASIONS

Abrasion wounds are the result of friction applied approximately parallel to the external surface of the skin. This friction usually results in the removal of variable amounts of the epidermis, dermis and hypodermis. In small animal practice these wounds are commonly seen as a result of road traffic accidents, for example where the animal has become trapped between the road surface and the moving vehicle. Such wounds are consequently frequently heavily contaminated with foreign material and bacteria and the frictional nature of the injury means that the bacteria and debris from the road surface are deeply embedded within the upper layers of the wound, therefore requiring careful debridement during the initial phases of wound management to ensure that all such debris has been removed from the wound. Abrasion wounds may also be seen as a result of poorly fitting casts and bandages, or from the abnormal wear of the patient's pads following prolonged contact with rough surfaces.

The effective debridement of these wounds is of paramount importance. As previously mentioned the debris from the road surface is often deeply embedded within the wound. These wounds are often located on the distal limbs, resulting in reconstruction being challenging, with skin grafting or open wound management being the only options for closure.

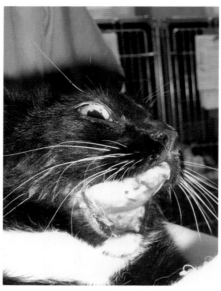

Figure 2.1   Feline patient post-road traffic accident with a degloved mandible

DEGLOVING WOUNDS

Degloving injuries are caused when the skin is torn from the underlying tissues, usually from a limb or occasionally the mandible (see Fig. 2.1).

Mechanical degloving occurs where the overlying tissue is torn from the sub-dermal plexus, e.g. following road traffic accidents. Physiological degloving occurs when the skin is sheared from the subcutaneous tissues therefore resulting in damage to the local blood supply and ischaemia of the area; this results in necrosis and sloughing of the skin over the following days. Secondary bacterial contamination frequently occurs with this physiological sloughing.

These injuries are relatively free from bacterial contamination following the initial injury, however during the sloughing process, which may take place over several days, secondary infection of the necrotic tissue may occur and hence problems will arise. The main problem with degloving injuries is the fact that large tissue deficits frequently result, particularly on the distal limbs, which makes reconstruction particularly challenging.

AVULSION INJURIES

Avulsion injuries refer to the forcible separation of tissues from their underlying attachments. Avulsion injuries frequently occur following dog bite wounds or road traffic accidents where the skin and subcutaneous tissue are avulsed from the mandible, resulting in the exposure of the underlying bone.

Again, the treatment and reconstruction of avulsion injuries pose the same challenges as degloving injuries, in that the injuries often result in large tissue deficits. However, bacterial contamination of avulsion injuries which arise as a result of dog fights are frequently heavily contaminated with bacteria, which make the initial treatment protocols vitally important in terms of reducing the bacterial load of a wound and the subsequent outcome of wound healing.

SHEARING

Shearing injuries have a similar aetiology to degloving wounds; they represent a combination of degloving and abrasion injuries and are frequently seen following road traffic accidents, with the wounds usually located on the patient's distal limb, particularly on the medial aspect of the carpus, phalanges and tarsometatarsal joint.

Shearing injuries tend to be deeper than abrasion injuries and may involve the underlying joints. Like abrasion injuries, large areas of tissue may be involved and will be heavily contaminated with foreign material, e.g. gravel and bacteria.

Shearing wounds tend to be extensive, deep and as a result a prolonged period of open wound management is often necessary (see Fig. 2.2). There may also be concurrent damage to the underlying joints and supporting soft tissue structures (tendons and ligaments) which may require external support of the joint during this period and ultimately prostheses and replacement of ligaments.

In severe cases, maintenance of joint function is not possible and therefore arthrodesis (surgical fusion of a joint) must be performed (see Fig. 2.3). In more severe cases, salvage of the limb is impossible and amputation will be necessary.

As with degloving and abrasion injuries, shearing injuries are commonly heavily contaminated with bacteria and debris from the abrading surface, e.g. a road. These wounds are therefore highly prone to infection and will frequently require long-term open wound management in order to overcome and prevent this. The decision between open wound management and reconstructive surgery is often dependent on the level of bacterial contamination within any joints which have been involved in the injury.

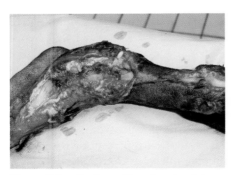

Figure 2.2   Canine with a shearing injury due to a road traffic accident

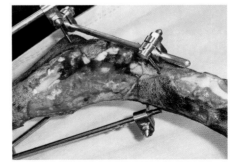

Figure 2.3   The same patient, now with the wound cleaned and debrided and after placement of an external fixator for treatment of orthopaedic injuries

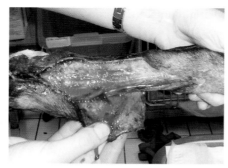

Figure 2.4 Incisional wound caused by glass

INCISIONAL

These wounds are most commonly seen in practice as surgical wounds but they can also be caused by trauma (see Fig. 2.4). In traumatic wounds the sharp object may be a piece of glass or a metal shard moving in a plane parallel to the skin surface. These wounds typically have clean, regular edges, which will gape open because of the inherent elasticity of the adjacent skin.

There is often relatively little involvement of the skin on either side of the wound, but the incision itself may be long and there may be extensive damage to the deeper tissues, e.g. muscle and tendons, nerves and blood vessels, which may not be detected on first inspection. This highlights how important it is to explore these wounds surgically for signs of further damage.

Contamination of such wounds is likely to be less than for abrasions. In addition, sharp trauma results in more bleeding, which will have an irrigating effect, thereby reducing contamination.

These wounds may be suitable for debridement and primary closure. However, delayed primary closure may be preferable if the wound is more than a few hours old or contamination is a concern. It should always be remembered, however, that the full depth of any wound should be explored prior to closure in order to ensure that there is no trauma to deeper structures, which may otherwise go unnoticed.

PUNCTURE WOUNDS

Puncture wounds are caused by a sharp object, e.g. a stick or metal railing (see Fig. 2.5), moving in a plane perpendicular to the skin surface. Penetrating wounds refer to those which have an entrance wound only, whereas perforating injuries refer to those with both an entrance and an exit wound.

Animal bite wounds, in which the skin is punctured primarily by the canine teeth of the aggressor, are the most common puncture wound seen in small animal practice. However, the puncture wound, which is often the most obvious manifestation of the trauma, is not the only consideration. Bite wounds often exhibit the 'iceberg' effect, where there is only a small surface wound but great underlying tissue damage.

The mobile superficial layers of the skin may be subjected to a laceration injury, as well as the puncture wound, and the deeper, more fixed tissues may be subject to crushing from the teeth. If the bite wound has been inflicted by another dog, the powerful masticatory muscles have the potential to crush tissues with a force of 150 to 450 psi, with the tips of the canine teeth puncturing and lacerating the skin (Swaim & Hendreson 1997). Movement and shaking actions will result in additional tears and avulsion of the tissues from their attachment to deeper structures, possibly resulting in devitalisation of tissues and the contamination of the wound with bacteria, deep into the subcutaneous and muscle tissues, predisposing bite wounds to infection.

All bite wounds therefore should be considered as contaminated wounds; if these wounds are left untreated, or are not treated using appropriate methods, the wound may become colonised by pathogens which may ultimately lead to an infected wound. Many clinical texts classify a wound as infected when the bacterial load of the wound is greater than 10^5 bacteria per gram of tissue (Slatter 2003).

The penetrating teeth force superficial tissue, including hair and bacteria from the aggressor's oral cavity, deep into the traumatised tissues. This results in a closed wound, which has no natural exit drainage route. Combined with the devitalised tissue and serum accumulation in the wound, this all provides an excellent culture medium for bacteria, with both aerobic and anaerobic bacteria interacting synergistically, resulting in rapid infection. Abscess formation, particularly in cats, may result in osteomyelitis of the underlying bone, therefore correct exploration and selection of antibiotic is of great importance.

Stick injuries should always be taken seriously as they may involve damage to the oesophagus or trachea, and as a result of the penetration the wound may extend down to the mediastinum which will be heavily contaminated by bacteria (see Fig. 2.6).

Firearm injuries and snakebites are also technically puncture wounds, but have additional complications over and above the initial puncture wound (see Figs 2.7 and 2.8).

Puncture wounds are generally treated by lavage using copious volumes of lactated Ringer's solution, debridement and drainage. Puncture wounds which arise as a result of animal bites generally have pockets of dead space which should be flushed and a dependent drain placed (see Fig. 2.9). It may also be worth obtaining a bacterial swab which may be sent to a laboratory for culture and sensitivity testing should wound healing not progress in a satisfactory manner. Dog bite wounds are generally allowed to heal by secondary intention using appropriate wound management dressings but, on some, occasional en bloc debridement may be performed in order to allow partial primary closure where there is sufficient tissue and skin available to perform this technique successfully.

Occasionally, dog bite wounds may not heal successfully and studies have indicated that this may be due to inadequate lavage, debridement and drainage, which highlights their importance in wound management.

Penetrating wounds to the thorax may result in rib trauma and pneumothorax and those to the abdomen may damage viscera. Penetrating bite wounds to the thorax which go unnoticed may eventually result in the formation of a pyothorax.

Snakebites

Snakebites are a particular subset of puncture wounds, complicated by the injection of the snake's venom. The adder is the only venomous snake found naturally in the UK and snakebites are occasionally seen in dogs exercised outdoors on areas of heath or moorland; in other countries there are a large variety of poisonous snakes found in both urban and rural areas. The snake's venom results in local and systemic effects. Local effects cause tissue necrosis and damage to blood vessel walls leading to ischaemia and tissue sloughing which may require skin reconstruction.

Snake venom results in the destruction of blood vessel walls which allows the leakage of blood into the surrounding tissue. Snake venom may additionally result in coagulation defects. The pain which is associated with snakebites may subside after 1–2 hours, when the tissue swelling and necrosis has an anaesthetic effect on the damaged tissue. The full extent of tissue damage will vary with the depth of the bite as well as the quantity of venom injected.

Local signs of snakebites include one or two fang puncture wounds (which may be bleeding), immediate or progressive swelling, tissue discolouration including petechiation and ecchymosis formation, as well as immediate pain.

The severity of snakebite signs will depend greatly on the quantity of venom injected and its location, and the tissue type (fat, muscle, etc.) in which the venom has been injected. The severity of the bite cannot be judged by local signs alone.

Systemic effects of snakebite include hypotension, shock, lethargy, salivation, painful lymph nodes, weakness, muscle twitching, and respiratory depression.

Early management of snakebite includes immobilisation of the affected part, by the application of a Robert Jones type dressing or splint, where possible, and avoidance of excitement or exertion during transit to a veterinary practice.

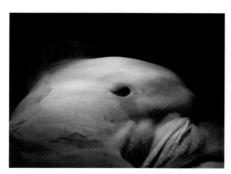

Figure 2.5   Entry wound from a bullet, over left scapula

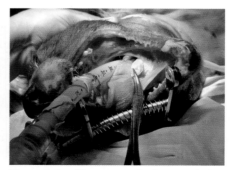

Figure 2.6   Placement of a Penrose drain in a patient following exploration of a stick injury. The wound beneath this patient's tongue was closed to allow dependent drainage of the tract, caused by the stick, at the exit point of the drain in the patient's throat

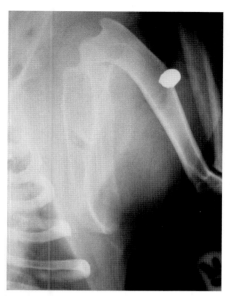

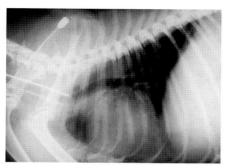

Figure 2.8 Radiograph demonstrating the bullet, from the patient in Figure 2.5, in situ

Figure 2.7 Radiograph demonstrating the bullet, from the patient in Figure 2.5, in situ

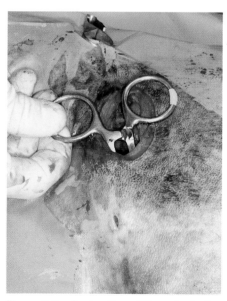

Figure 2.9 Exploration of the extent of damage of puncture wounds

These wounds usually involve an extremity or the ventrum. The wound is usually grossly swollen and initially oedematous. Later there is progression to ischaemia and necrosis of large areas of tissue around the site of the puncture.

BURNS

These wounds can result in both local and systemic complications, including the loss of a large area of skin, and wound infection (see Fig. 2.10).

Systemic complications include hyper-/hyponatraemia, hyper-/hypokalaemia, metabolic acidosis, pre-renal azotaemia, anaemia and septicaemia.

Burns are often extensive and reconstruction of the large skin deficits often presents a challenge, however their occurrence is very rare in small animal practice. Eschar formation invariably results in large tissue deficits; it is important to remove this eschar (the slough or dry, black scab which forms following a burn injury) in order to get back to a healthy granulation bed. Secondary bacterial contamination is common in burn wounds but septicaemia is uncommon.

Burn wounds are generally classified according to the method of infliction, the depth of the injury, or the surface area involved. Burns are also further classified into partial thickness or full-thickness injuries.

First degree, or superficial burns, affect only the epidermis. Following the injury the dermis becomes very thickened and erythematous. First degree burns can take 3 to 6 days to heal, by the process of re-epithelialisation, and the regrowth of hair at the site is likely.

Second degree, or partial thickness burns, involve both the epidermis and varying amounts of the dermis. Such burns result in subcutaneous oedema and a marked inflammatory response. These wounds heal by re-epithelialisation from the remnants of the deep adnexa. The rate of wound healing and the return of hair growth are dependent upon the extent and depth of the burn.

Third degree, or full thickness burns, result in the destruction of the entire skin thickness. These burns result in the formation of an eschar, which is the dark brown, insensitive, leathery covering of the damaged skin. With third degree burns the superficial subcutaneous blood vessels are thrombosed and the deeper blood vessels become highly permeable, which results in oedema in the subcutaneous tissues and necrosis of the damaged tissue. With these types of burns the true extent of the burn may not be initially obvious, with the the damage extending far beyond the initial area.

Superficial burns will often heal by secondary intention, but partial thickness burns may result in significant scarring with possible compromise of function if the burn is situated close to a joint or natural body orifice (e.g. mouth or anus). Full thickness burns will require surgical reconstruction, i.e. flaps or grafts.

Burns may be thermal (hot or cold), chemical (acid or alkali), electrical or radiant in origin.

Thermal burns

These are caused by extremes of temperature, generally heat rather than cold. Hyperthermic burns may be caused by exposure to hot water (scald), contact

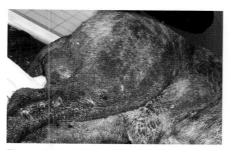

Figure 2.10   This patient had been thrown into a refuse chute which had been set alight; this photograph demonstrates the injuries due to plastic melting onto the patient's skin

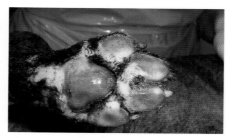

Figure 2.11   The same patient, showing burns to the pads of the feet

with hot surfaces, e.g. car exhaust during road traffic accidents, or exposure to burning materials.

Iatrogenic burns

One cause of thermal burns can be the use of electrical heating pads placed under an animal, particularly during or after anaesthesia or in reptiles lying on a heat mat or beneath a heat lamp which is not connected to a thermostat to regulate heat output. Burns from external heat sources are more likely if the heat mat is used for prolonged periods or at too high a temperature in recumbent patients who cannot change position. Animals with poor cutaneous blood flow arising from hypothermia may be at particular risk.

Hypothermic burns

Hypothermic burns may result from exposure to a cold environmental temperature, i.e. frostbite. Environmental hypothermic injury usually affects the extremities, such as the toes, tail and ear tips, but damage as a result of contact with cold objects may affect any part of the body. Hypothermic injuries are not commonly seen in the UK.

Chemical burns

Chemical burns are caused by exposure to acid or alkali. These wounds often involve the pads (see Fig. 2.11), although oropharyngeal burns may occur in cases of ingestion. This type of burn may also be caused maliciously.

Electrical burns

Electrical burns may be direct (contact) burns, where the animal touches, or more commonly chews through, a low tension electrical source, such as domestic electrical cables, or indirect (flash or arc burns) where the animal comes too close to a high tension electrical source, e.g. railway lines.

Contact burns result from the current passing through the body and are often caused by the animal chewing through an electrical cable.

Radiation burns

Radiation burns may be caused by exposure to sunlight (sunburn) or radiation machines. They may result from doses greater than 40–50 Gy, depending on the radiation tolerance of the exposed tissue and the nature of the radiation.

MANAGEMENT OF BURN WOUNDS

Thermal burns

In terms of proposed treatments and recovery rates of burns patients, it is advisable that treatment is commenced for all patients suffering first degree burns and for those patients with second or third degree burns which do not cover more than 50% of the patient's total body surface area. In patients who suffer partial or full thickness burns to more than 50% of their body, euthanasia should be considered or referral for specialist treatment offered.

Burn wounds can be very difficult to detect in small animals as they do not always blister; in addition, a thick coat may cover the burn. Within a few hours of the injury there will be the development of erythema (reddening of the skin), transudation of fluid, and easily epilated hair follicles (hair which can easily be pulled out).

The ultimate depth and extent of tissue injury may not be readily apparent for 24–72 hours, at which time obvious margins of demarcation between healthy and non-viable tissue usually develop.

Temperatures which can result in thermal injuries do not need to be excessively high, as the extent of tissue injury is dependent upon both the temperature and the length of exposure. Thermal injuries have been seen at temperatures as low as 44°C (111°F) with prolonged exposure, e.g. such injuries are all too often seen in patients placed on heat mats during surgery, as a result of the use of hot hair dryers and because of poorly earthed diathermy units.

Hospitalised animals frequently have underlying conditions which predispose them to thermal burns. The ability of an animal to dissipate heat from an area of local application can affect the extent of the injury. Animals with poor peripheral perfusion, e.g. shocked or hypothermic patients, or patients that are dehydrated are at an increased risk when they are exposed to relatively low-temperature heating devices (42°C) for prolonged periods of time.

In order to prevent such iatrogenic thermal burns from occurring, patients should not be placed on electrical heating sources, e.g. heat mats; if possible circulating warming devices should be used, which use either water or air (BairHuggers™) to gently warm the patient or maintain body temperature whilst under GA (general anaesthetic).

TREATMENT OF BURN WOUNDS

With immediate burns treatment should be commenced, if possible by the owner, with the application of towels soaked in ice water or the submersion of the area in cold water; this will help to relieve pain and arrest the progression of the burn.

If hair still remains over the burned skin, the depth and extent of the burn may be estimated by pulling the hair from the skin. If this is easily done then this suggests the burn is full thickness. Any remaining hair and surrounding hair should be clipped and the area washed in dilute antiseptic.

Loose debris and necrotic tissue of the surface of the skin should be removed when the cleansing of the wound takes place.

Full-thickness burn wounds should be aggressively debrided as soon as areas of non-viable tissue are established. Maintaining the eschar over a burn wound is contraindicated and is associated with an increased risk of infection and wound complications. Debridement can be conservative (hydrotherapy, wet dressings) or aggressive via surgical debridement techniques. In second degree burns eschars should be debrided to the point where petechial bleeding is seen. Third degree burns should have the eschar surgically removed as soon as possible as it may retain infection beneath it. The wound edges should be splinted, therefore preventing wound contraction. As the eschar separates away from the underlying tissues, it should be gently removed using scissors.

Dressings for burn wounds depend upon the size of the wound and any accompanying systemic factors. Smaller burn wounds in patients that are systemically healthy can be dressed with wet-to-dry dressings as part of the debridement process. Larger wounds in a debilitated patient should be dressed with non-adherent contact dressings which provide a moist wound environment. Topical non-irritating antimicrobial (water miscible) agent, such as silver sulfadiazine, is useful.

Daily inspection and redressing of the wounds is generally required for the first few days as progressive tissue injury can occur during this period. The wound should be gently lavaged using lactated Ringer's solution of sodium chloride 0.9% solution. Debridement should be repeated as necessary in order to remove all non-viable tissue before the dressings are replaced.

Superficial burns should heal well via open wound management, as the wound will heal by re-epithelialisation.

Partial thickness burns may also heal by open wound management which will result in a thinly haired scar, or it may be preferable to remove the scar tissue and then close the wound surgically if the defect is not too large as this may give a more cosmetically pleasing result.

Full thickness wounds are more difficult to treat and should be reconstructed as soon as:

- there is no ongoing tissue necrosis
- all non-viable tissue has been debrided from the wound
- there is no complicating wound sepsis
- in many cases this may be as early as 2–3 days post-injury.

In considering the management of wound reconstruction various factors need to be taken into consideration in order to select the optimal method for reconstruction. Options include:

- mesh grafts
- axial pattern flaps
- skin advancement.

Immediate treatment of severe burn wounds in canine and feline patients

Intravenous fluid therapy should be commenced immediately, using a balanced electrolyte solution. A concurrent reduction in intravascular fluid volume must be offset in order to maintain cardiac output and peripheral tissue perfusion. Colloid and plasma replacement therapy is generally not indicated for the first 24 hours following injury as the continuous escape of large-molecular weight compounds through damaged vessel walls may exacerbate ongoing fluid shifts. Analgesia must be provided, in the form of opioids; the use of NSAIDs (non-steroidal anti-inflammatory drugs) is controversial – they will reduce the extent of ongoing tissue injury, but it is important to ensure adequate renal function prior to their administration. Topical cooling is also effective in reducing pain associated with burn wounds.

Burn patients should be fed at least 1.5 times their resting energy requirement. One major problem is that many burns patients will not eat following injury, particularly if oropharyngeal oedema is present. In such cases the placement of oesophagostomy or gastrostomy tubes may be indicated.

Electrical burns

Low tension electrical burns occur when an electrical current touches one point on the body with or without points of exit. This is most commonly seen when animals chew on electric cables. The point of contact with the current is usually charred, but the electric current may then flow along blood vessels, resulting in thermal damage within the vessel and surrounding tissues supplied by the blood vessel. On initial inspection, immediately following the injury, the tissue may appear undamaged; however, ischaemic demarcation and sloughing will occur in 2 to 3 weeks.

Following electrical burns to animals' mouths and lips, the tissues should be observed regularly for a 2- to 3-week period, with the debridement and removal of devitalised tissue as necessary. By the end of the 2- or 3-week period most of the devitalised tissue should have separated and the full extent of tissue damage will be known. At this point any resulting defects may be reconstructed as necessary (see Fig. 2.12).

Chemical burns

Such burns can be caused both accidentally and maliciously. They arise following contact with oxidising agents, reducing agents, corrosives, etc.; such agents result in the denaturation and coagulation of tissue protein. Treatment is similar to that for thermal burns.

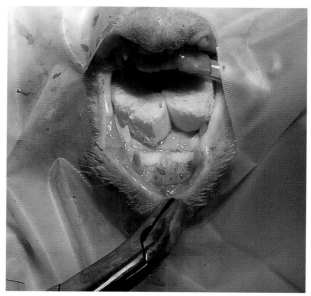

Figure 2.12   Feline patient undergoing a mandibulectomy and maxillectomy after chewing through an electrical cable. The devitalised bone can be seen clearly, as the injury resulted in the loss of the patient's lower incisors, 2 weeks following the injury, as well as necrosis of the surrounding tissues

Initial treatment of such burns involves the rapid dilution of the chemical agent by repeated lavage of the area with copious quantities of water; this will assist in the removal of the chemical agent and its dilution, therefore hopefully reducing its chemical reaction with the animal's tissues. It is also vitally important to prevent the animal from interfering with or licking the burned area as this may result in burns to the oropharynx and oesophagus.

Following repeated lavage, treatment should continue as for thermal burns. This will include:

- removal of devitalised tissue
- topical application of an antibacterial agent and appropriate dressing
- daily dressing removal and continued tissue debridement as required
- re-application of medication and dressings, with appropriate changes as wound healing progresses.

Once all devitalised tissue has been removed and a healthy granulation bed is present the decision can then be made on whether to treat via open wound management or to close the defect with a skin flap or graft.

The initial treatment in terms of debridement of chemical burns can be difficult. If the wound debridement is too conservative and the wound is not debrided early enough, then this may result in further tissue destruction secondary to continued chemical penetration. This will be seen 24 to 72 hours post-injury. However, aggressive early debridement may result in the removal of too much tissue and hence make healing or closure of such wounds prolonged and difficult.

FIREARMS INJURIES

The response of tissues to ballistic injuries is complex. The basic wound is a perforating or penetrating injury, but with extensive damage to the underlying tissue as the projectile moves on its trajectory.

The bullet will cause stretching, compression and laceration of tissue. Slow velocity entry wounds are typically small, but the exit wounds may be large. Damage to tissue along the path of the projectile is likely to be more severe than the cutaneous wound. The pattern of trauma is determined by the velocity of the missile. As velocity increases then the kinetic energy imparted to the tissues increases exponentially. Shotguns, airguns and handguns are classed as slow velocity (where the bullet travels at less than 1000 feet per second). As the projectile passes through the tissues it results in a permanent tract by crushing, lacerating and damaging tissues in contact with the missile. Low velocity projectiles generally result in small entry and exit holes, but the resulting tract will have bacterial contamination. Deeper tissues are damaged by a compression wave which moves ahead of the bullet and it is this compression wave which damages the tissues.

High velocity gunshot wounds usually result from rifles; the bullet travels more than 2000 feet per second. They result in a greater amount of tissue damage and transfer considerable energy to the adjacent tissues in the form of shock waves and cavitation. It is the shock wave that causes blunt contusions of the associated tissues; this momentary stretching and tearing of vessels which occurs results in haemorrhage and thrombosis. As with low velocity wounds, the projectile will result in the implosion of debris into the wound and the resulting contamination. All these factors result in infection, with the severity of necrosis dependent on the severity of the vascular compromise. High velocity gunshot wounds frequently result in orthopaedic fractures, bowel ruptures and cardiac and pulmonary contusions due to the shock waves, without these organs ever being in direct contact with the missile.

Gunshot wounds are still fairly uncommon in veterinary practice but their occurrence is ever increasing. It is worth considering the possibility of gunshot wounds with any puncture wound, but they may be the result of various types of ballistics. The obvious appearance of superficial pellets, the combination of a small entry wound and much larger exit wound, extensive subcutaneous emphysema, bloodstained fur and often abnormal posture or limb function due to pain, may indicate a shooting.

The entrance wound may be difficult to find, especially with smaller projectiles. Extensive shaving of the fur may be required to identify the wound. The presence of fur drawn into the wound is almost always diagnostic.

On radiography, the situation is almost always obvious (see Fig. 2.13). However, high velocity projectiles, especially in small animals (particularly birds),

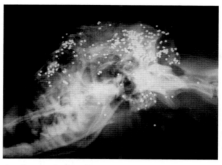

Figure 2.13   Radiograph of a patient taken postmortem in order to diagnose the cause of death which demonstrates the results of a shotgun wound

may pass through the body, leaving no trace, or often a small amount of metallic dust, especially if they hit bone.

In rifle injuries, it is the pressure wave that causes most of the damage, rather than the bullet itself. This cavitating effect, in the wake of the bullet travelling at supersonic speeds, causes massive tissue disruption, to a diameter of 6 to 12 cm in standard rifle rounds.

It is important to consider where pellets have gone on their passage through the body. Once they are identified on radiography, and localised (which may be much more difficult than one would expect) the pathway should be checked for debris sucked in by the projectile creating a vacuum as it travels through the tissues, and thoroughly lavaged and debrided. The placement of a Penrose drain may also be indicated. This feature is most pronounced in high velocity projectiles.

There is an argument for leaving many projectiles in place if there appears to be no associated infection or foreign body reaction, and many animals radiographed for other reasons reveal clinically silent pellets.

CAST AND BANDAGE WOUNDS

Any bandage or cast must be checked daily by the owner who should always be provided with a written information sheet featuring a checklist of points for examination. The bandage or cast should also be examined by a veterinary surgeon on a regular basis and replaced if there are any doubts about its suitability.

Iatrogenic wounds caused by poorly fitting casts and bandages are important and can potentially result in serious injuries.

Loose bandages or casts may result in abrasions or ischaemia secondary to pressure over bony prominences.

The distal limb, especially its focal pressure points, e.g. the olecranon or os calcis, is usually involved. These wounds are caused by a combination of poor bandaging and poor owner compliance and veterinary management of the patient.

PRESSURE SORES (DECUBITUS ULCERS)

These are open wounds which develop over bony prominences due to pressure in recumbent animals. These sores develop due to pathological changes in soft tissues caused by their compression between bony prominences and the surface on which the animal is resting (see Fig. 2.14).

The areas of skin most subject to pressure sores are those over the ischiatic tuberosity, greater trochanter, tube coxae, acromion of the scapula, lateral epicondyle of the humerus, lateral condyle of the tibia, lateral malleolus, lateral aspect of digit five, olecranon, calcaneal tuber and sternum.

The main therapy is the prevention of pressure over the ulcer. This can be achieved by the form of a pressure relief bandage, e.g. a doughnut bandage or foam padding, over the affected area. This must be dressed carefully in place to prevent the dressing slipping and resulting in further areas of pressure necrosis.

Ultimately, it is the prevention of such pressure sores that is important, ensuring the patient is placed on well padded bedding, e.g. water or air beds or acrylic bedding.

EXAMINATION AND ASSESSMENT OF THE WOUND

When a patient which has sustained some type of wound is presented to the surgery, it is the initial examination and assessment for treatment which frequently fall to the veterinary nurse in the 'triage nurse' role.

Initial assessment and treatment is an extremely important phase of wound management as it is the most critical step in controlling wound contamination and maximising host defences. These two processes are essential to the prevention of wound infection. Wound infection is the most devastating factor to impede wound healing and any effort to prevent wound infection, as opposed to attempting to treat wound infection, is extremely important.

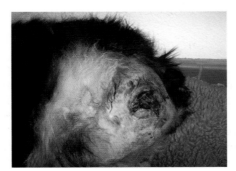

Figure 2.14   An extensive decubitus ulcer present over the ischiatic tuberosity in a canine patient

The initial examination needs to include an assessment of the patient as a whole. Many wounds are the result of trauma; there may be concurrent injuries which may be of more importance in the initial stages, e.g. pneumothorax, etc. It is essential that the patient is stable before any detailed wound management is carried out. The provision of analgesia is also required at this stage in the form of opioids and possibly non-steriodal anti-inflammatory drugs; this is not only essential for ensuring the patient is more comfortable but will also make the clinical examination possible and less painful for the animal.

A full history and thorough clinical examination is necessary in order to anticipate complications which may affect the wound healing process. A history of any medication which the patient may be receiving should be noted, as this may affect the healing process, e.g. corticosteroids.

Once the patient is stable a more detailed examination of the wound can be performed and wound cleaning carried out. Effective cleaning of the wound may require sedation or a general anaesthetic, particularly if the wound is painful, e.g. extensive shearing injuries involving a joint.

If it is anticipated that a wound will require prolonged treatment and repeated dressings which may require sedation, or general anaesthesia will be necessary, then the owner should be advised on the likely outcome of the wound and an estimate of the likely costs should be made, as this can very quickly become extremely expensive.

If during the initial treatment of a wound, the patient is deemed too high a risk for a general anaesthetic, topical lidocaine (lignocaine) 2% may be applied to the wound, combined with some sedation and analgesia, to make the cleaning of the wound more comfortable for the patient. The lidocaine (lignocaine) may be applied by placing a soaked gauze swab on the wound for several minutes or via injection through intact skin around the periphery of the wound. Lidocaine (lignocaine) containing vasoconstrictors, i.e. adrenaline (epinephrine), should not be used as this would reduce the blood supply to the area and ultimately affect wound healing.

FACTORS TO CONSIDER AND ASSESS ON INITIAL PRESENTATION

Bacterial contamination

The only wound which can be classed as truly clean is a surgically made one, where bacterial contamination has been strictly controlled and minimised via correct preparation of the environment, i.e. properly cleaned theatre, skin preparation with suitable antimicrobial agents with the correct contact period, sterile consumables, etc.

The neutrophils in the initial clot and inflammatory fluid will be the first line of defence against bacterial proliferation. If this defence is overwhelmed, the wound will become infected. Toxins released by the bacteria and cell lysis will cause erosion of the wound bed, inhibiting the development of wound strength and delaying contraction and epithelialisation.

The optimal time for treating an open wound is thought to be within the first 6 hours (the 'golden period') at which point the wound is considered contaminated, but not infected. A figure of up to 10^5 bacteria/g of tissue has been proposed as an indication of wound infection. However, the degree to which this principle holds depends on the circumstances under which the wound was created, including the degree of trauma and the amount of foreign material present. Clinically, small numbers of bacteria in a deep ischaemic wound may be more significant than higher numbers in an open draining wound with healthy granulation tissue. Bite wounds have a great potential for delayed necrosis and infection, not only due to the contamination but also the crush and penetrating injuries sustained by the patient.

Viability, type of tissue and vascular supply

The blood supply to the wound is vital to allow access for cells necessary for debridement and defence. Consequently, in devitalised tissue, healing is delayed and the likelihood of infection is increased but also large areas of devitalised or necrotic tissue will be isolated from the immune defences of the patient and therefore will be more susceptible to bacterial proliferation and invasion. Crush injuries have extensive subcutaneous bruising predisposing them to infection in the necrotic or ischaemic tissue, which acts as a perfect culture medium for bacterial growth. Likewise, if the vascular supply is compromised by swelling or laceration of major vessels, bacteria will be able to invade the tissues. Shock will result in peripheral vasoconstriction; if the circulation is not regained, a relative ischaemia of wounds of the peripheral limbs may be seen.

The ability to resist infection varies according to the type of tissue. Well vascularised areas of skin will tend to have good bacterial defences whereas fat or structures such as joints have poor defences. Oral wounds heal surprisingly well due to the vascularity of the mucosal epithelium.

All devitalised tissue (including blood clots, skin and hair fragments, tissue desiccated by exposure, and plugs of tissue resulting from ligation or diathermy of bleeding vessels) has to be degraded and phagocytosed by macrophages before healing can progress. Haematomas are inaccessible to the body's defence systems and are likely to become infected.

Foreign material

All foreign material has to be removed before the wound will be able to heal. However, the system can cope better with less antigenic particles, such as sand, than with clay soil particles or organic debris. The presence of foreign material that cannot be removed by macrophages is associated with sinus formation, chronic wound infection and prolonged healing times. Ballistic wounds result in a tract of debris through the tissues which compromises healing and requires aggressive management. Shear injuries of the distal limb, commonly seen in road traffic accidents, have foreign material ground into the bone and soft tissues and therefore require extensive debridement and lavaging (see Fig. 2.15).

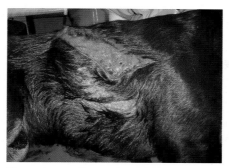

Figure 2.15   Contaminated wound
post-road traffic accident

WOUND CONTAMINATION CLASSIFICATION

Wounds can be classified by their level of 'contamination'; the following groups
are generally used:

Clean wounds

These are wounds which have been created under sterile conditions, which do
not enter into any of the following body cavities: gastrointestinal, respiratory,
genitourinary or oropharyngeal. As a result, clean wounds are limited to those
created during surgical procedures, e.g. mass removal.

Clean–contaminated wounds

These are wounds which have minimal contamination, and the level of contamination can be removed or reduced to a biologically insignificant level. Surgical
wounds involving the gastrointestinal, respiratory, genitourinary or oropharyngeal cavities may be considered clean-contaminated wounds. Wounds which
have been created under traumatic conditions should not be classed as clean-
contaminated upon initial presentation, but it may be possible to convert such
wounds to a state considered clean-contaminated through lavage and debridement.

Contaminated wounds

These are wounds which are heavily contaminated; they frequently include wounds
which have foreign matter present. Surgical procedures which feature a major
break in aseptic technique (such as the spillage of gastrointestinal contents during
an enterotomy) or acutely presented traumatic wounds are classed as contaminated.

Dirty wounds

These are wounds in which active infection is present, such as an old traumatic
wound with purulent exudate or perforated viscus.

In general, all traumatic open wounds are classed as contaminated or dirty at the time of initial presentation, and such wounds can never be converted to a clean state. The closure of such wounds should only ever be considered once the wound has been converted into a clean-contaminated state, and this is following lavage and debridement and possibly a period of open wound management.

Most wounds may be converted from a clean-contaminated to a dirty state, if there is no ongoing tissue necrosis, within 72 hours of injury, if aggressive and appropriate wound management is used.

MANAGEMENT OF THE WOUND

The aim of wound management is to optimise the conditions for wound healing. Depending on the wound, this may mean preparation for primary closure or temporary decontamination and debridement until closure is possible or healing has occurred. The first stage is decontamination as far as possible, given the state of the wound and the condition of the patient; this also encompasses prevention of further contamination in the hospital or by the animal. The second stage is debridement of necrotic or devitalised tissue and removal of any foreign debris. The final result should be control of infection and establishment of a healthy wound bed enabling closure of skin deficits.

SKIN PREPARATION

The aim of skin preparation is to prevent further contamination of the wound. Wounds in loose skinned areas may be protected by temporary closure with towel clips, continuous suture or by stapling. Large wounds or wounds in areas where the skin is under tension may be packed with sterile swabs or a water soluble jelly during clipping and cleaning. The clipper blades must be disinfected and without missing teeth that may further traumatise healthy skin. Hair at the edges of the wound may be trimmed with scissors wetted or dipped in water soluble jelly so that the hair sticks to the blades and does not fall into the wound. When a wide area around the wound has been clipped, the jelly or swabs and clipped hair are removed and replaced with fresh sterile swabs to protect the open wound while the surrounding skin is prepared with surgical scrub solutions. Ideally, all staff should wear sterile gloves throughout this procedure to prevent the further contamination of the wound with the operator's commensal skin bacteria.

Alcohol should never be used as part of skin preparation as it may result in delayed healing times.

Lavage

The aims of lavage are to remove gross debris and to dilute bacterial contamination. Initially, gross contamination or necrotic tissue may be simply washed away gently with tap water, using a hand shower. Afterwards, the wound is lavaged more carefully. The wound should be treated in a sterile manner to prevent further contamination and the clean area surrounding the wound should be protected or re-scrubbed, as necessary.

Choice of lavage solution

The ideal lavage solution is lactated Ringer's solution. This is used in large volumes to dilute and wash out bacteria and debris without causing any physiological damage to the normal cellular processes within the wound bed. There is little justification for the use of antiseptics in the lavage of moist open wounds; the effectiveness of wound lavage has been shown to be proportional to the volume of fluid used, suggesting that dilution, rather than bactericidal activity, is of great importance. Copious gentle lavage using isotonic solutions, together with careful wound debridement, is the ideal (Fowler & Williams 1999).

Sodium chloride (0.9%) has always been thought to be a suitable lavage solution; however studies have indicated that this may exert cytotoxic effects as it does not contain a buffer and also has an acidic pH. However, if lactated Ringer's solution is unavailable then normal saline would be the next most suitable alternative (Fowler & Williams 1999).

Antiseptic solutions may have a place in the management of severely infected wounds, where necrosis and lysis are more significant than the proliferation of host cells, as well as in patients that are immunosuppressed and hence at greater risk from infection. Antibiotics have also been added to lavage solutions, especially in anaerobically infected wounds. Soluble antibiotics such as metronidazole, penicillins and neomycin may be used but it is questionable whether the antibiotic will reach a sufficient concentration for a long enough period of time to have any bactericidal effect. Antiseptics or antibiotics should never be used as a substitute for good surgical debridement and aseptic wound management techniques.

All substances added to a lavage solution have the potential to damage not only the bacteria but also the host's cells. Antiseptic solutions, therefore, must be used at the correct concentration. This means a 0.05% solution of chlorhexidine gluconate (Hibiscrub™, Mallinckrodt), which is the equivalent of 1 ml to 80 ml. In very necrotic or purulent wounds, repeated lavage will be necessary to gain the benefits of the bactericidal action of the antiseptic.

Hypochlorite (Dakin's solution), hydrogen peroxide and cetrimide/chlorhexidine (Savlon™ Veterinary Concentrate, Mallinckrodt) have all been used to irrigate wounds. These solutions are irritant and highly toxic to the host cells and therefore should not be used for wound lavage.

Irrigation pressure

The suggested pressure for the irrigation is 8 psi in order to lavage a wound adequately, which may be achieved using a 20-ml syringe with an 18 gauge needle or catheter attached at an angle of 45° (see Fig. 2.16). Higher pressures may force contamination deeper into the wound or cause oedema in adjacent tissue. The patient should be protected from becoming soaked and the wound should be allowed to drain freely.

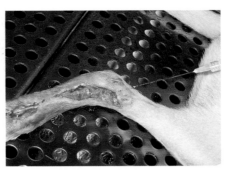

Figure 2.16   Lavage of a shearing wound

Lavage alone is not sufficient to allow wound closure or decontamination. The next stage of wound management is debridement.

Debridement

The aim of debridement is to remove all tissue which is thought to be devitalised, contaminated or infected as well as removing embedded foreign material from the wound. This allows rapid onset of the proliferative phase of healing, by reducing the amount of debridement necessary by the macrophages in the wound bed. Removal of this material also assists in the control of infection and also enables the surgeon to explore the full extent of the injury and any damage to underlying structures. It is the single most important step in the management of a wound and is often performed inadequately.

Good wound debridement will involve a combination of methods and procedures in order to convert the wound into a surgically clean wound. If there is doubt as to whether tissue is viable, the wound should be debrided in stages over a period of a few days. A contaminated wound can potentially be converted into a surgically clean wound by one-stage debridement. An infected wound will require staged debridement to achieve a surgically clean wound.

If there is any doubt as to the viability of tissue at the time of injury then it is best to repeat debridement conservatively, and opt for open wound management. In this situation the wound can be assessed, lavaged and debrided once or twice daily until the extent of tissue necrosis is controlled. If necessary, open wound management should be performed for 2–3 days prior to wound closure.

Surgical debridement

Surgical debridement is the best way to remove grossly contaminated tissue in order to prepare the wound for suturing, or as part of a staged procedure of selective debridement of non-viable tissue. A sharp scalpel blade (not scissors) should be used for incisions and lavage may be repeated as debridement progresses (see Fig. 2.17).

The wound should be draped and prepared as for surgery to minimise iatrogenic contamination. As debridement progresses, the surgical instruments should be changed, to prevent contamination of clean areas. Sensitive, gentle handling of viable tissue is essential for achieving a healthy wound. Skin edges should be protected or handled with skin hooks; bent 20 gauge needles are suitable. Retractors should not be used. Haemostasis is important to prevent haematoma formation and the separation of wound surfaces. However, plugs of necrotic tissue from electocautery or multiple ligatures can also delay healing as well as acting as a focus for infection.

Surgical exploration of the wound will enable visualisation of local anatomical structures to check that they are unaffected. An apparently simple, small laceration near the stifle could hide a deep puncture wound involving the joint which may severely affect the prognosis. The exploration should be extensive enough to establish the limits of the wound without risking contamination of unaffected tissues or disruption of the fascial planes of tissue that are natural barriers to bacterial invasion.

En bloc debridement This technique is generally indicated for infected wounds where there is no vital tissue involved and where there is sufficient skin to allow reconstruction. The wound is packed with surgical gauze swabs and then closed, retaining the swabs within the wound. The whole area is then excised as one piece, as with the removal of a mass, with a margin, hence preventing the contamination of the surrounding tissues. Once this has been performed the remaining skin deficit is then treated as a clean surgical wound which may be closed routinely.

Layered debridement This involves the gradual removal of devitalised tissue, layer by layer, thereby allowing the conservation of healthy tissues where possible, which may be reassessed at a later date for further debridement if this is thought necessary. This debridement technique is particularly useful for lesions on the limbs or feet where excess skin is not available, and conservation of vital structures is extremely important. The technique may be used where the removal of grossly contaminated or necrotic tissue may be necessary; the surgery may be followed by the application of debridement dressings, with daily inspection to allow reassessment and hence saving viable tissues as much as is possible.

Once the wound has been surgically debrided as much as is possible, the decision needs to be made as to whether to close the wound or continue debridement using other techniques. If there is any doubt as to the viability of a wound, a debriding dressing should be placed and the wound then reassessed 24 hours later.

Non-surgical debridement

Debridement dressings Such dressings allow further debridement of the wound after surgical excision of grossly devitalised tissue has been completed. These dressings are especially useful in encouraging rapid establishment of granulation tissue in the management of wound healing by second intention and also allow debridement of contaminated or infected wounds.

The primary dressing layer is an adherent open weave mesh (sterile surgical swab), which is protected by standard secondary and tertiary bandage layers. This

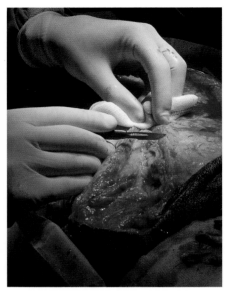

Figure 2.17   Manual debridement prior to wound closure

mesh traps debris and necrotic tissue which is then removed at each dressing change (see Fig. 2.18). A 'dry-to-dry' dressing (dry mesh gauze) is occasionally indicated where there is a profuse low viscosity exudate. For a 'wet-to-dry' dressing, the gauze is applied moistened with sterile saline or lactated Ringer's solution. Wet-to-dry dressings can be useful for gently debriding excessive granulation tissue, or restimulating chronic granulation tissue. Additionally, any wound that is purulent, malodorous or slow to heal, with retreating epithelial edges, may benefit from 1 to 3 days of wet to dry dressings in order to restimulate healing. Adequate debridement in this way often controls bacterial infection in the wound more effectively than high dose antibiotic therapy. Wet-to-dry dressings are not used on exudate wounds, as they can macerate the tissues and cause more damage. It is vital that these dressings are changed daily, in order to prevent desiccation or maceration of the wound as well as to ensure that the dressing performs its function effectively.

Enzymatic debridement   This involves the use of enzymes (e.g. streptokinase and streptodornase powder [Varidase™, Lederle]) to break down and allow the removal of necrotic tissue without disrupting or slowing the development of normal granulation tissue. The process is slow, but will preserve structures that are healthy and vital, such as nerves. These dressings must be changed daily, which may prove expensive if extensive debridement is necessary. The enzymes will also erode healthy tissue, hence these dressings must be used with great care and stopped once granulation tissue has been established. The use of such agents has generally been overtaken by the use of the hydrogels.

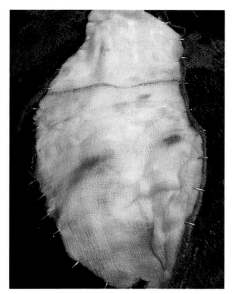

Figure 2.18   Placement of a wet-to-dry dressing in the patient in Figure 2.16

Debridement cream or solution

Dermisol™ (SmithKline Beecham) is a mixture of dilute acids (benzoic acid and malic acid) and propylene glycol in a cream or solution. It debrides the wound by differential swelling of healthy and necrotic tissue, which is achieved by the solution having a low pH. Its main use is in the early management of contaminated wounds. It is toxic to healthy granulation tissue and is indicated only in the early management of wounds. It is generally not recommended that such debriding solutions be used at all due to their acidity as well as the availability of more suitable agents.

Other agents

These include products such as hydrogen peroxide and wound powders, which have no role in wound management and therefore should never be used. Hydrogen peroxide only acts to damage cells, particularly those in the capillary bed, and hence results in a significant delay in the wound healing process. Wound powders simply act as foreign material when they are placed within a wound and hence result in delayed healing times as they must be cleared by inflammatory cells before healing can progress; they may also predispose to foreign body granuloma formation.

Debridement of different tissue types

Skin – immediate assessment of viability may be misleading due to vascular spasm. The skin edges should be trimmed carefully, removing only non-viable portions of skin; staged debridement should be considered if there is any uncertainty as to the viability of the skin, in order to allow the recovery of as much skin as possible. One useful tip is to draw the outline of the area of skin which is thought to be non-viable; this may be done using a sterile surgical pen, so that accurate reassessment can be made at a later stage. This method also ensures that non-viable portions of skin are not included in the closure of a wound which may become necrotic, resulting in further surgery at a later date and consequently increased costs for the client, not to mention further procedures for the patient.

Fat – all exposed fat should be debrided to a clean non-necrotic plane.

Muscle – muscle which appears dark, friable or fails to contract should be debrided. Muscle ischaemia causes cell death within 4 hours, so again it may be useful to consider staged or delayed debridement.

Nerves – nerves should be conserved and protected from other damaged tissue wherever possible.

Joints – should be lavaged thoroughly and repaired where possible.

Tendons – again should be preserved as much as possible. If infection is present then any anastomosis of tendons will fail and any repairs to tendons will take 3 to 5 months to develop strength.

Ongoing care of the wound

Once debridement has been performed and the wound has been converted to a 'clean' wound by lavage and debridement, the decision must be made as to whether or not to close the wound. For both the surgeon and the owner the most satisfactory outcome arises from primary closure, and this is generally the most common method for surgical wounds. However, due to the nature of the injury and the extent of the damage, for many traumatic wounds this technique is not initially an option, hence the decision must be made as to 'when' the wound should be closed.

In order to close a wound the following criteria must be fulfilled:

- There should be sufficient tissue to allow the reconstruction of the wound without dehiscence (breakdown)
- The wound should be free from foreign material or devitalised tissue
- There must be no sign of infection or contamination
- The surrounding skin must be healthy and viable.

OPTIONS FOR MANAGEMENT OF AN OPEN WOUND
Primary closure

A typical example of a wound which is suitable for primary closure is a clean surgical wound where the surrounding skin and tissues are brought into close apposition by sutures or staples and healing of the wound is expected to take place, with minimal scarring, within 10 days.

With some non-surgically created wounds it still may be possible to perform primary closure if decontamination, via lavage and debridement, is satisfactory, although it may be necessary to place a drain, e.g. dog bite wounds.

Delayed primary closure

Delayed primary closure is performed in order to allow the staged debridement of the wound for 2 to 3 days. Once early granulation tissue has begun to form, this generally indicates that the wound bed is free from infection and hence the wound is at a suitable point for surgical closure.

Secondary closure

This type of closure is performed in wounds with more extensive tissue damage and where there may be the presence of a bacterial infection. In such wounds, several days of wound debridement may be required, hence allowing the development of a more mature granulation bed before surgical closure is performed. Once the wound reaches this stage, contraction of the wound will also have commenced, therefore incision and undermining of the granulation bed must be performed in order to allow the release of the skin from the wound bed and the advancement of the skin over the wound. When secondary closure of a wound is completed the wound may exhibit greater strength due to the granulation tissue underlying the wound, however the wound may demonstrate reduced mobility.

Healing by secondary intention

When a wound is allowed to heal by secondary intention, the wound is left to granulate, contract and epithelialise without any surgical intervention. This technique involves debridement of the wound until there is a healthy granulation tissue bed with epithelialisation from the skin around the wound edges. Such wounds require repeated dressings which will retain moisture within the wound, allow rapid epithelial migration and proliferation, whilst also keeping the granulation tissue bed healthy and protected.

Antibiotic therapy

Traumatic wounds are generally considered contaminated on initial assessment, and therefore the administration of systemic antibiotics should be considered in order to reduce the rate of invasion of bacteria, with intravenous or intramuscular preparations being ideal, rather than any 'long acting' subcutaneous preparations. The antibiotic may not reach therapeutic levels in severely traumatised tissue so other methods of reducing the level of contamination, e.g. lavage, debridement and placement of appropriate dressings, should be commenced. A broad spectrum antibiotic with low systemic toxicity and good tissue penetration is indicated. It is vital that the correct dose rate (according to the animal's body-weight) is calculated and administered at an interval frequent enough to maintain a therapeutic concentration of the antibiotic over each 24-hour period.

Bite wounds are usually infected with *Pasteurella* species, and ampicillin or amoxicillin are suitable first line antibiotics. Other types of skin wounds may be contaminated with staphylococci or *Escherichia coli* and amoxicillin (amoxycillin)/clavulanate, trimethoprim/sulphonamide combinations or cephalosporins are indicated. Metronidazole or clindamycin may be selected if there is a suspicion of an anaerobic infection, but this must be used in combination with another broad spectrum antibiotic. Fluroquinolones should not be used as a first choice antibiotic for a minor infection sensitive to β-lactam antibiotics.

Culture and sensitivity tests should be performed if the patient shows systemic signs of sepsis or the wound is exudative and lytic or 'melting'. The initial choice of antibiotic may be governed by the availability of an intravenous veterinary preparation. A rough estimation of the type of contaminant can be made by making an impression smear from the wound and performing a Gram stain on it in order to make an appropriate choice of antibiotic.

MANAGEMENT OF TRAUMATIC WOUNDS

The majority of traumatic wounds are not life threatening, but the animal's initial assessment and treatment may ultimately determine the final outcome of such wounds. The incidence of healing complications and pain may be minimised by accurate surgical management which at the same time may improve the chances of a satisfactory outcome.

When dealing with small wounds it is not uncommon for them to heal relatively quickly despite poor wound management. However, if the same approach is applied to larger wounds this may result in complications in the healing process, e.g. dehiscence or infection, and these factors may result in compromise of limb function due to extensive tissue loss and even amputation of the limb.

Some wounds may be allowed to heal via secondary intention; such wounds include:

- Those without major tissue loss
- Wounds which are free from large areas of necrotic tissue
- Wounds which are confined to non-vital areas
- Wounds which are open to drainage
- Wounds which are not overwhelmed by pathogens and contaminants
- Wounds where secondary intention healing and scarring will not affect joint movement
- Where leaving a wound to heal by secondary intention will not cause pain or suffering.

For wounds which are more serious and extensive, where gross contamination is present, and where there is necrotic tissue and insufficient drainage, appropriate and effective treatment is critical to the welfare of the patient and the ultimate outcome of the wound.

The healing and outcome of a wound is dependent upon the careful application of appropriate techniques, attention to detail and strict adherence to the principles of wound management.

Triage assessment of wounds

Veterinary nurses are frequently in the frontline when dealing with wounds in an emergency situation, or offering telephone advice to clients at the scene of the accident. Owners need to be told to deal with the patient gently in order to minimise stress in an already frightened patient. The owner should also be told to muzzle the patient where suitable and appropriate, as these patients, no matter how stoic in everyday life, may bite when moved or handled.

When offering telephone advice to a client it is best to recommend to cover the wound in order to prevent further contamination; this is best done using sterile moistened gauze, but in an emergency situation a piece of clean moistened linen is best applied to the open wound. This will act to prevent the wound from further trauma, prevent contamination, patient interference and also to encourage haemostasis.

It may be necessary for pressure to be applied if an arterial bleed is suspected. Clients should never be told to apply a tourniquet as incorrect use may cause further and more severe trauma as a result of ischaemia.

If a fracture is suspected, additional support may be required; this may be achieved with the application of a firm bandage or splint, which will help in the reduction of pain and may help reduce further soft tissue injury. If an open fracture is present the application of a dressing would help in the reduction of contamination of deeper tissues.

If spinal injury is suspected then the patient should be transported on a flat surface, e.g. the parcel shelf from a car.

Initial wound assessment and dressing placement

The nurse assessing the patient needs to ensure that a full history is obtained, to include current medical problems and any medication currently being used. The cause of the wound should also be established so the treatment can be tailored accordingly, e.g. the treatment of dog bite wounds will differ from wounds sustained from broken glass.

A full evaluation of the patient should also be made, ensuring that an adequate airway is present and that the animal is breathing normally and the patient's circulation should be assessed by thoracic auscultation and palpation of the patient's pulses. If any of the above are of concern the triage nurse should then take appropriate measures as necessary in order to stabilise the patient.

A detailed physical examination should then be performed, with an assessment of any problems detected, and further examination of the wound should be made.

If definitive wound management is likely to be delayed then action should be taken in order to prevent further deterioration and contamination of the wound. A swab of the wound should be taken for bacterial culture, so appropriate antibiosis can be selected and a sterile dressing, plus a support dressing where necessary, should be applied. In the interim the veterinary surgeon may wish to commence some antibiotic therapy and analgesia should be provided, ideally in the form of non-steroidal anti-inflammatory drugs (NSAIDs) and opioids as deemed necessary.

Wound evaluation

The nature and extent of the wound needs to be established, i.e. the situation under which the wound was created and the extent of tissue damage. The remainder of the affected region of the body must also be examined for further less obvious signs of damage which may be overlooked in the haste of dealing with the more obvious problems.

Wounds which are overlying the thorax or abdomen need to be examined carefully and thoroughly; the pleural and peritoneal spaces need to be examined in order to ensure that they are intact and there are no signs of pneumothorax or penetrating abdominal injury. In practice, ideally all animals should have routine thoracic and pelvic radiographs taken following RTAs (road traffic accidents) to eliminate any life threatening injuries.

For wounds which are located on the limbs, damage to the underlying bones, joints and underlying neurovascular structures should be ruled out.

The aim of initial wound management is to encourage the development of a healthy vascular wound bed, which is free from necrotic tissue, debris and infection.

Prevention of further wound contamination

Once the patient has been admitted to the surgery, action needs to be taken to ensure the wound is protected from any further contamination, particularly from nosocomial infections, trauma or desiccation, by covering the wound with a sterile dressing. If debridement of tissues is necessary then the use of saline soaked gauze swabs, i.e. wet-to-dry dressings, are useful. It should also be reiterated that ideally sterile surgical gloves should be worn when dealing with wounds in practice and the increasing incidence of cases of MRSA in veterinary practice only goes to highlight this point.

Occasionally some veterinary surgeons will use antiseptic solutions to soak these dressings, e.g. 0.05% chlorhexidine gluconate or 1% povidine iodine solution. The use of such solutions is questionable as many initial dressings are used to debride contaminated or necrotic tissue and any infection detected is generally controlled with the use of systemic antibiotics. Once the required amount of tissue has been debrided then the resulting granulation tissue is generally resistant to infection.

In order for wounds to be correctly debrided and dressed, general anaesthesia or sedation will be necessary. If the patient is thought to be too high a risk for such sedation then it may be necessary to apply local anaesthetic directly to the wound as a 'splash block' or infiltrated around the wound bed. If this is not possible then a regional nerve block may be indicated. The use of lidocaine (lignocaine) and adrenaline (epinephrine) may be contraindicated as blood flow to the wound bed may be reduced.

The area surrounding the wound needs to be clipped so that the wound can be adequately cleaned without contaminating the wound further; the exposed surface of the wound should be protected by either filling the wound with water-soluble gel, e.g. KY Jelly™ or hydrogels, e.g. intrasite gel, or by the placement of saline soaked swabs covering the wound (see Fig. 2.19). This is done to prevent debris and clipped hair fragments from entering the wound. A generous amount

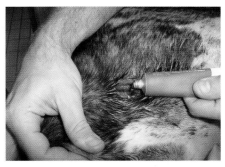

Figure 2.19   Placement of water–soluble gel in a wound to prevent further contamination during clipping and cleaning of the wound

of hair, approximately 20-cm margin, is clipped around the wound. The gel or swabs are then removed and the surrounding skin is then aseptically prepared as for surgery.

Wound debridement

All necrotic tissue needs to be removed from the wound to allow healing to occur. Areas in which the tissue may be of questionable viability may be excised if not essential to normal function, e.g. subcutaneous fat, or if there is any concern staged debridement may be performed, particularly if the tissue is surrounding structures necessary for normal function, e.g. tendons.

Any necrotic tissue, particulate debris and micro-organisms will encourage infection and delay the process of healing. At this stage a bacteriology swab should be taken in order to assess the contaminants present.

Any tissue which may be grossly contaminated should be removed by debridement. Other tissues should be debrided via mechanical debridement, i.e. physical removal of the debris followed by pressure lavage using an isotonic solution, e.g. saline or lactated Ringer's solution, in order to removal any contaminants left behind following mechanical debridement.

Large volumes of fluids are required in order to lavage the wound adequately. A simple technique for the rapid lavage of such wounds is to connect a 20-ml syringe to an 18 gauge needle via a three-way tap and a giving set; this system results in pressure irrigation at 8 psi, which is considered ideal for the dislodgement of debris, bacteria, and devitalised tissue. The fluid can then be flushed over the surface of the wound, at an angle of approximately 45° in order to prevent pushing debris deeper into the wound. The wound edges should be gently lifted in order to examine the deeper tissue planes. If any debris is present then these deeper tissue planes can also be lavaged. With puncture wounds, e.g. dog bite wounds, any pockets of dead space should be repeatedly lavaged and will greatly benefit from flushing and dependent drainage.

Further debridement of the wound can be performed following the initial stage of wound management with the application of wet-to-dry dressings. This is the moistening of surgical swabs with sterile saline; these swabs are then applied to the wound bed and covered with dry swabs and then cotton wool and held in place with bandages.

The moist swabs will dry onto the wound bed and adhere to the surface. When they are removed, the action of removal will mechanically debride the wound. This debridement process will remove necrotic tissue, debris and other contaminants.

A viable vascular bed is crucial to the effective healing of the wound. Wound management aims to promote the improvement of the patient's circulation to the wound, but at the same time reducing the potential for infection and other adverse consequences of wounding.

Bandages are used to protect the wound from contamination and trauma and limit oedema.

References and further reading

Anderson D 1996 Wound management in small animal practice. In Practice 18(3): 115-128

Baines SJ 2003 Aetiology of cutaneous wounds. Veterinary Times Dec 2003: 8-10

Fowler D, Williams JM 1999 Open wound management. Manual of canine and feline wound management and reconstruction. BSAVA, UK

Hayes G, Yates D 2003 Understanding dog bite wounds. Veterinary Times Nov 2003: 16

Saunders R 2004 Ballistic injuries of animals. Veterinary Times Nov 2004: 8-10

Slatter D 2003 Textbook of small animal surgery. WB Saunders, Philadelphia

Swaim SF, Henderson RA 1997 Specific types of wounds in small animal wound management, 2nd edn. Williams and Wilkins, Baltimore

Chapter 3
The process of wound healing
Louise O'Dwyer

Wound healing is a complex process and the treatment of the wound will depend on the stage of healing, therefore it is important that veterinary nurses fully understand the processes which are occurring during each phase of healing so that the treatment can be tailored to gain the best outcome. This chapter will identify the processes which are occurring during the different stages.

Wound healing can be described as the physiological process of restoring the continuity of the tissues following injury. Wound healing can be divided into two main processes: regeneration and repair.

Regeneration is the replacement of the lost cells or tissues with normal functioning cells of the same type. Only tissue or organs that maintain a cell population capable of undergoing mitosis, such as epithelia, bone or liver, are able to heal in this way. If this process is not possible then in most mammalian tissues the healing will occur by repair. This is the formation of a relatively avascular, collagen-rich scar which holds the adjacent edges of the wound together.

Normal wound healing occurs as a continuous event, which may be divided into three different phases:

The inflammatory (or substrate) phase (immediate)
The proliferative (or repair) phase (days 3 to 7 post-injury)
The remodelling (or maturation) phase (days 5 to 7 onwards following injury).

Each of the above phases do not occur at completely separate times as completely separate processes, but in fact all three processes overlap and therefore ultimately influence the development and duration of the next phase, meaning each individual phase is critical to the final result.

The importance of the wound healing phases in any particular wound may vary depending upon the individual wound environment, and is generally dictated by wound factors (e.g. nature of the wound, degree of contamination) and host factors (e.g. patient health status, immunosuppression, age).

Normal wound healing is a highly organised and complex cascade of biochemical and cellular events which, hopefully, will result in a successful outcome. However, should one of the phases of healing be prolonged or fail then this may result in the failure of wound healing.

The damaged tissue is disorganised, hypoxic and contaminated with debris and dead cells. Neutrophils are the predominant cell 8 to 18 hours after injury. They debride the wound, kill bacteria and stimulate the arrival of other types of cells.

PHASES OF WOUND HEALING

1. INFLAMMATORY PHASE

Main features of this phase of wound healing:

- Wound retraction
- Haemostasis
- Increased vascular permeability
- Migration of leukocytes
- Wound debridement.

Early inflammatory phase

The initial injury triggers coagulation and stimulation of the inflammatory cascade resulting in chemotaxis and an influx of inflammatory cells; the magnitude of this inflammatory response will be dependent on the severity of the trauma.

Wound retraction

Immediately following the initial wounding, the tissue defect tends to enlarge due to the normal tensions present within the tissues (this can be seen when any surgical incision is made) and, in some cases, the direct action of muscle fibres that attach to the skin.

Haemorrhage

Trauma to the blood vessels within the wound results in haemorrhage. This haemorrhage has beneficial effects in that it helps to clean the wound and starts the process of allowing the cellular and humoral components of the healing process to arrive at the wound surface.

Haemostasis

Within a few minutes of the wounding, vasoconstriction mediated via catecholamine release, limits haemorrhage from small vessels and lasts for 5–10 minutes. This is followed by the aggregation of platelets to exposed sub-endothelial collagen and the formation of a primary platelet plug, which is stabilised into a secondary plug by clotting factors later in the process. Injured cells release thromboplastin, which activates the extrinsic coagulation process.

Advantages of the clot

- Haemostasis
- Prevention of further wound contamination
- Prevention of wound dehydration
- Initial fibrin network for cellular migration.

Disadvantages of the clot

- Increased quantity of cellular debris that must be removed in later phases of wound healing
- Enlargement of the dead space
- Provision of a medium for bacterial growth.

At the surface of the wound, the clotting cascade results in the formation of a clot, which, on exposure to air, dehydrates and contracts, forming a scab. The scab has a number of useful functions:

- Prevention of further haemorrhage
- Protection from external contamination
- Maintenance of the wound microenvironment
- Provision of a surface below which epithelial cell migration can occur.

The scab does not provide any wound strength and eventually sloughs, together with dead bacteria and leukocytes.

Inflammation

After 5–10 minutes, the inflammation phase proper starts, with vasodilation and increased vascular permeability.

The classic signs of inflammation, i.e. heat, redness, pain and swelling, are seen at this time and are due to:

- Vasodilation
- Extravasation of fluid
- Obstruction of the local lymphatic channels
- Stimulation of local nerve endings by pressure, stretching and chemical stimulation (e.g. bradykinin).

Debridement phase

The main features of this phase are:

- Migration of leukocytes
- Removal of cellular debris
- Phagocytosis and killing of bacteria.

A number of different cell types enter the wound during the debridement phase. Their relative contribution changes with time and the need for their particular function. The removal of necrotic tissue is essential for the healing process to continue.

Cell types involved in the debridement phase of wound healing include:

- Neutrophils
- Platelets
- Monocytes/macrophages
- Lymphocytes.

Within 30–40 minutes of injury, the vessel endothelium at the site of injury is coated by leukocytes, particularly along the venules. Polymorphonuclear neutrophils are the first cells to arrive, followed by the mononuclear cells, monocytes and lymphocytes.

Neutrophils

Neutrophils enter the wound within 6 hours of injury and increase to maximum numbers over 2–3 days.

Neutrophil chemoattraction is mediated by:

- Signals from damaged endothelium
- Release of fibrinopeptides as fibrinogen is processed into fibrin
- Production of proteinases by neutrophils degrading necrotic tissue.

The role of the neutrophil is to destroy bacteria, either by phagocytosis and intracellular destruction or by extracellular killing by liberation of hydrolytic enzymes, such as elastase and collagenase, from their granules. The presence of these enzymes in the interstitial space aids in the removal of damaged tissue and cellular debris. In the absence of infection, the number of neutrophils decreases rapidly. If there is no bacterial contamination, wound healing may still occur in the absence of neutrophils, since their phagocytic function may be performed by macrophages. The combination of wound fluid, degraded neutrophils and denatured tissue constitutes the exudate seen at this time, referred to as pus.

Platelets

Platelets are the first cells with a reparative function to enter the wound and play an important role in haemostasis. Platelets produce a number of growth factors which act as chemoattractants and proliferative factors for other cell types.

Growth factors produced by platelets include:

- Platelet-derived growth factor (PDGF)
- Epidermal growth factor (EGF)
- Platelet factor IV
- Insulin-like growth factor (IGF-1)
- Transforming growth factor β (TGF-β)
- Endothelial chemoattractive factor.

Bacterial products also act as chemoattractants for leukocytes.

Monocytes

Monocytes leave the circulation to enter the wound and become macrophages. Monocytes play an essential role in wound healing. Absence of the other cell types involved in wound healing will still result in wound healing, although this may be at a slower rate, but in the absence of monocytes, the wound will not heal. Macrophages are present within the wound 1–2 days after injury.

Initially monocytes enter the wound with neutrophils in the same proportion as their relative proportions in peripheral blood, and neutrophils predominate. However, as the inflammatory phase progresses, monocytes are actively recruited via a cytokine released by activated cells in the wound, extracellular matrix degradation products and other inflammatory mediators. In addition, monocytes are relatively long-lived compared to neutrophils and, as time progresses, macrophages become more numerous than neutrophils.

Macrophages play a vital role in wound healing, particularly in governing the transition from the inflammatory phase, and have a number of different roles:

- Phagocytosis and killing of bacteria
- Debridement of the wound by phagocytosis and release of enzymes (e.g. collagenase)
- Regulation of the synthesis of intercellular matrix
- Control of cell recruitment and activation
- Stimulation of angiogenesis.

Lymphocytes

Lymphocytes play a role in the innate and adaptive immune response to foreign antigens and microorganisms. Antigen presenting cells, including macrophages and dendritic cells, present antigens to lymphocytes thus initiating an immune response; they do have a positive effect on the rate and quality of tissue repair.

The extravasated fluid, cells and dead tissue comprise the inflammatory exudates seen in the wound at this time. As the neutrophils accumulate, die and undergo lysis, the exudate becomes purulent. As the debridement phase wanes, the exudate reduces in quantity.

Severe tissue trauma resulting in vascular compromise will result in reduced circulation and will cause a reduction in the local tissue pH from lactic acidosis. This environment favours the release of proteolytic enzymes from the breakdown of local connective tissue and allows the inflammatory reaction to spread, potentially forming an abscess.

As the inflammatory phase wanes, local vascular permeability is restored and the extravasation of leukocytes into the wound is reduced. If an agent capable of inciting inflammation, such as foreign material or bacteria, is present in the wound, monocytes undergo local proliferation, which is a characteristic of chronic inflammation.

Granulation tissue formation

The result of fibroblast proliferation and capillary ingrowth is the production of granulation tissue, which is composed of capillary loops capped by fibroblasts and macrophages. The presence of the capillary loops give the tissue a granular appearance, hence the name. Granulation tissue typically appears by day 3–6 after wounding (see Fig. 3.1). In small wounds, this tissue will lie beneath a scab.

Granulation tissue is important for the following reasons:

- It is resistant to local infection by microorganisms
- It serves as a barrier to systemic infection
- It provides a surface over which epithelial cells can migrate
- It plays a role in wound contraction
- It contain the fibroblasts that produce collagen
- It provides an excellent blood supply for wound healing by other methods, e.g. secondary closure, free skin grafts and pedicle flaps.

Thus, in the management of any open management of any open wound which is not suitable for primary closure or delayed primary closure, the formation of a healthy bed of granulation tissue should be regarded as the initial goal, from which decisions regarding further closure options may be made.

Resistance to infection

Healthy granulation tissue is highly efficient at fending off bacterial infection. This resistance is due to the recruitment of inflammatory cells in the first phase

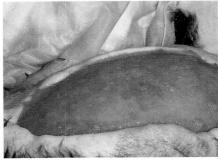

Figure 3.1   A healthy granulation bed

Late inflammatory phase

Macrophages infiltrate shortly after inflammation is established and are crucial to the stimulation and progression of the wound through the phases of the healing. They debride necrotic or foreign material in the wound and dispose of the platelet clot, dead cells, bacteria and organic debris. Macrophages are derived from the circulating monocytes and are stimulated by factors such as endotoxins, alginate, cytokines, fibrin, hypoxia and increased lactate concentrations. In monocytopaenic patients, this stage is delayed or fails altogether.

Activated macrophages release growth factors and enzymes which stimulate or inhibit other cells in the healing wound. Maximal stimulation of macrophages can be a disadvantage – a heavily contaminated wound may remain in the inflammatory phase, delaying healing and creating more scar tissue.

2. PROLIFERATIVE PHASE

This phase comprises three main events:

Proliferation of fibroblasts and collagen synthesis
Proliferation of endothelial cells and infiltration of capillaries
Proliferation and migration of epithelial cells.

The transition from the inflammatory phase to the production of granulation tissue occurs at 3–5 days after injury and the first 3–5 days are sometimes referred to as the lag phase of wound healing. It is important to realise that this represents a lag in the gain of tensile strength, not a lag in wound repair.

The proliferative phase marks the development of granulation tissue. Fibroblasts migrate into the wound from nearby skin. They lay down a new extracellular matrix after debridement has taken place, and manufacture and remodel collagen. Fibroplasia is almost entirely dependent upon the inflammatory trigger and may be delayed if the inflammatory phase fails to occur. However, once the fibroblast population is active and in place, anti-inflammatory drugs will not halt the formation of normal scar tissue.

Fibroblasts start to lay down collagen 4 to 5 days after injury. This is dependent upon a well oxygenated environment and good nutrition. In a hypoxic environment, the formation of normal collagen fails to take place, and therefore good vascular perfusion is required for normal wound healing. Collagen production is poor in diabetic patients or those with cardiovascular disease.

Excess lactate, synthesised by the macrophages, also stimulates collagen depo-

of wound healing and non-specific antibacterial processes, together with the good blood supply and oxygenation of fresh granulation tissue.

Wound contraction

In loose-skinned areas, wound contraction can account for up to 30% of closure of a skin deficit. The process is due to active contraction of myofibroblasts and manipulation of collagen molecules laid down in the wound. A greater degree of contraction is seen in burn wounds or infected wounds where the extracellular matrix is extensively degraded. Contraction can result in loss of function if it occurs over a joint or body opening.

3. REMODELLING PHASE

This phase consists primarily of:

- A balance of collagen deposition and collagenolysis
- Remodelling of the collagen molecules, fibres and bundles
- Regression of the vascular elements.

This final phase is the remodelling and restoration of the normal structure. The scar, however, will nearly always be weaker than the surrounding uninjured skin.

Once collagen is laid down, lysis and reformation take place rapidly and persistently. Any normal wound will break down if the collagen reformation slows while lysis continues. Thus, the nutritional needs and oxygen supply to the wound are critical to wound strength even after the first few days. Infection results in delayed healing due to the release of toxic metabolites. This causes collagen and matrix lysis and loss of mass. In the initial stages, if the inflammatory, debridement and proteolysis are proceeding at a greater rate than fibroblasts, the wound deepens and the tissue is digested.

MOISTURE BALANCE AND EXUDATE CONTROL

The wound healing process relies on the activity of:

- Cells, such as leucocytes, fibroblasts, endothelial cells and keratinocytes
- Protein, such as enzymes, growth factors and collagen
- Chemicals, such as oxygen and nutrients.

This activity during the healing process requires hydration. When a wound is sustained, extracellular fluid forms the basis of wound exudates which are modified by the process of inflammation. During the inflammatory phase of wound healing, histamines are released which act on the blood capillaries resulting in their increased permeability. Serous fluid and white blood cells begin to leak into the tissues, helping to maintain the moisture levels within the wound bed. The redness which occurs around the wound is the result of the engorgement of the capillaries being visible through the skin.

Wound exudates contain high levels of growth factors and cytokines, and products of the autolytic digestion of non-viable tissue and bacteria. As wound healing progresses, the level of exudate decreases.

An acute wound may fail to heal as a result of intrinsic factors, including:

- Immune-compromised patients
- Severe respiratory or cardiac disease
- Severe anaemia.

Or it may fail to heal as a result of certain extrinsic factors, such as:

- Excessive bacterial levels
- Excessive mechanical stress on the wound.

When this occurs, the composition of the exudates takes on the profile of a chronic wound.

A chronic wound requires constant reassessment, so as to identify the stage of wound healing correctly and select the best treatment. In a normal, acute healing wound the exudate will dry out to form a scab. This will re-establish the normal hydrostatic pressure within the wound bed, and form a barrier to bacteria. Wound healing will take place beneath the scab; however, in most wounds the scab restricts the migration of epithelial cells, and hence slows down the healing process. This can be avoided by dislodging the scab, although this action, in turn, exposes the wound to the air which in turn can delay wound healing as a result of dehydration. The use of wound dressings provides a moist wound environment which is optimal for wound healing; providing that the wound is constantly checked, reassessed and the wound dressing changed regularly.

Studies have demonstrated that large quantities of normal wound exudates are not harmful to the wound, but chronic wound exudates frequently contain high levels of proteases (tissue destructive enzymes) and these are associated with delayed healing.

The effect of wound exudates also needs to be considered in terms of the surrounding healthy, undamaged skin, as excessive exudate can cause maceration or excoriation resulting in skin breakdown and possible extension of the wound.

Regular changing of the dressing will also provide the clinician with a good opportunity to assess the colour and consistency of the exudates as this can provide information as to the cause and, therefore, the treatment or appropriate dressing required.

Dressings manage exudate in three ways:

- Absorption: based on the actual volume that the dressing can actually hold
- Evaporation: the transmission of water vapour through the dressing (this is dependent upon how porous or 'breathable' the dressing is)
- Hydrostatic pressure.

Choosing an appropriate dressing can be challenging and careful consideration needs to be paid to the dressing most suitable during each phase of wound healing to give the best possible clinical outcome.

EPITHELIALISATION

Full thickness wounds left to heal by 'secondary intention' go through three stages:

- Formation of granulation tissue
- Wound contraction
- Epithelialisation.

Epithelialisation is the process during which the germinal layer of the epidermis (*stratum basale*) responds to chemical signals to proliferate and migrate across the granulation tissue to form a new layer of epidermal cells.

Several factors must be present for epithelialisation to occur:

- There must be a good wound bed of well-vascularised granulation tissue and a supply of oxygen and nutrients from nearby capillaries. Epithelialisation will not occur across poorly-vascularised or necrotic tissue.
- There should be a low level of inhibitory chemical factors, such as toxin produced by certain bacteria (e.g. *Staphylococcus aureus*).
- There must be a source of viable epidermal cells. The source of these cells is normally the edge of the wound.

This last point highlights why particularly large ulcers and wounds take a particularly long time to heal, despite the fact that all other factors for healing are optimal. The progress of a healing wound can be represented by the change in size of the open part of the wound over time. This is possible due to the fact that as the new epidermis forms a new *stratum corneum*, fluid loss is reduced and the dry epithelial edge becomes visible. The final phase of healing can therefore be represented by the change in size of a wound over time.

The speed of wound healing can be accelerated by the use of skin grafts which reduce the size of the wound as well as providing an additional source of viable epidermal cells. The success of skin grafting relies heavily on the presence of a healthy granulation bed on which the skin graft can 'take'. The skin graft also needs to remain immobile on the wound surface for a long enough period of time to adhere and to acquire a new blood supply, hence this is not a procedure suitable for use in wounds which have become infected or necrotic.

Further reading

Anderson D 1996 Wound management in small animal practice. In Practice Mar 1996: 115-128

Baines SJ 2004 Wound healing and reconstructive surgery. Part 1: Anatomy of the skin. UK Vet 9(7): 22-30

Baines SJ 2005 Normal wound healing. UK Vet 10(6): 16-28

Chapter 4

Open wound management

Louise O'Dwyer

If a wound is unable to be surgically closed then it will be necessary for the wound to heal by secondary intention. Open wound management is a technique which provides the ideal environment for rapid and successful wound healing. However, the choices in wound dressings available on the veterinary market can be very confusing for the veterinary nurse and surgeon. This chapter aims to categorise the different primary layer dressings available into:

- Adherent vs. non-adherent
- Occlusive or permeable
- Interactive/bioactive or non-interactive.

These categories will cover the dressings available, their differences and their indications and aims. This section will also discuss other dressings which may still be used in general practice but which are now outdated and should not be used, and discuss the reasoning behind this. There will also be a section devoted to newer and alternative methods of treating wounds such as honey, enzymatic debridement, aloe vera and larval therapy.

All wound dressings are designed with a specific function in mind, and are aimed at a specific stage of the healing of the wound. Although protection of the wound is one of the reasons for their placement, their use may not be simply to prevent contamination but in fact to interact with the wound and promote rapid wound healing. This is the area in which the veterinary surgeon or nurse should have thorough knowledge in order to select the most appropriate type of dressing.

Bandages generally have three basic layers; this chapter will look at the choice of primary or contact layer dressings and how and when these dressings should be used.

A wound needs to be monitored closely to differentiate the changes as it progresses through the various healing stages. As this occurs, different dressings may become appropriate. Ideally, the animal should be hospitalised for the early part of the wound management process to allow the dressing to be changed as often as required (even two or three times per day or more often if, for instance, an animal urinates on the dressing). In general practice, this may be difficult but, in order to carry out effective wound management, bandages should be changed at least once per day, in the first few days. There are few bandages that can protect a wound for more than 2 to 3 days, particularly in the early stages of wound healing.

WHAT FACTORS DELAY NORMAL WOUND HEALING?

Anything that allows the inflammatory phase to persist will delay the normal healing process. Such factors may include infection, foreign material, desiccation and necrosis of superficial layers of tissue, and continuing tissue damage. All incite an inflammatory response and therefore delay the development of granulation tissue and hence, healing. Healthy granulation tissue is extremely resistant to infection – a patient with a healthy granulating wound does not need systemic antibiotic treatment. However, granulation tissue is susceptible to damage caused by abrasion, trauma, desiccation or chemical irritation (e.g. urine scald). It is therefore possible for a healing wound that was granulating, epithelialising and contracting to come to a grinding halt and turn into chronic indolent granulation tissue. It is important to recognise when this is happening and to know the most appropriate action to take in order to reverse the changes.

FACTORS WHICH PROMOTE HEALING

It has been demonstrated that optimal healing will occur under the following conditions:

- Moist local environment (but not so wet as to result in maceration)
- No infection/necrosis present within the wound
- No toxins/particles/loose fibres to contaminate the wound
- Optimal temperature (35–37°C)
- pH should be maintained at around 6, which helps to inhibit bacterial multiplication.

Therefore, treatment of any open wound must aim to:

- Prevent further tissue damage, including desiccation of the surface tissue (allowing a wound to 'dry out a bit' does not accelerate healing)
- Prevent any further contamination of the wound
- Resolve infection
- Remove all necrotic material and tissue.

Hence, the functions of veterinary wound dressings include:

- The debridement of any necrotic or infected tissue and assisting in the removal of any foreign matter within the wound which may inhibit healing processes and therefore healing
- The absorption of any exudate to allow healing processes to occur

- Providing protection of the delicate wound surface from the secondary layer of the dressing as well as trauma from the patient or the environment
- Prevention of infection or strike-through of the bandage and hence the migration of bacteria through the dressing and onto the wound
- Provision of analgesia
- Encouragemnet of wound healing by creating the optimum environment
- Immobilisation of the wound surfaces, ensuring that the capillary buds and migrating epithelial cells are not disrupted, therefore maximising the rate of wound healing
- First aid: it can be used as a temporary first aid measure to protect the wound from further contamination and aid haemostasis while a trauma patient is stabilised. The wound should be covered with a non-adherent dressing and a secondary absorbent layer. At this stage, ointments, antiseptics or wound powders may result in chemical damage and complicate debridement later on.

It should always be remembered that the primary layer should always be sterile and should remain in close contact with the wound surface whether the patient is resting or moving. If there is any space present between the dressing and the wound this may result in reduced drainage from the wound and subsequent possible tissue maceration, as well as possible further wounds resulting from pressure and irritation from the moving dressing. It is therefore essential that the primary layer conforms well to the patient's contours (see Ch. 6). If a wound is present that is exudative or draining then it is essential that the contact layer will allow the fluid to pass through the dressing to the secondary or absorbent layer. Dressings placed on non-exudative wounds should prevent external contamination. Meshed materials should be fine enough to prevent penetration by fibrinous tissue. The contact layer should also minimise pain, prevent unnecessary loss of fluids and be non-toxic and non-irritating.

Wound dressings can be placed into several categories, with some more modern dressings encompassing more than one of these categories:

- Adherent vs. non-adherent
- Occlusive or permeable
- Interactive/bioactive or non-interactive.

We have already looked at how the treatment of wounds has changed through the years and the past 20 years has seen a massive range of wound dressings introduced to both the human and veterinary market and a general change in the use of active dressings over passive dressings to improve wound healing. In order to choose a dressing suitable for a particular type of wound and its stage in the healing process we firstly need to be familiar with the products available, the ways in which they work and their suitability.

All wound dressings have a specific function and are designed for use on a wound at a specific stage of healing, so no one particular dressing is suitable for all stages of the healing process. Several factors need to be taken into consideration when choosing a wound dressing:

- What is the plan for the treatment of this wound? Do we want to perform delayed primary closure, secondary closure or second intention healing? The new 'TIME' concept is very useful in aiding the selection of the most appropriate dressing – see later.
- The current stage of wound healing – inflammatory, proliferative or maturation phase. If there is the presence of granulation tissue the wound will require a dressing that will not disturb the delicate blood vessels and epithelial cells of the granulation bed. A wound at this stage will require the correct environment to allow the epithelialisation and contraction phases to occur with minimal disturbance, and ideally increase the speed at which this process can occur and produce a cosmetically satisfactory result.
- Is necrotic tissue, foreign material, infection or exudate present? This type of wound will require debridement and therefore the choice needs to be made as to the type of debridement which will be suitable, i.e. surgical, mechanical, chemical debridement, for the patient and for the owner in terms of cost and time taken up by dressing changes, etc.
- Is chronic granulation tissue present? If this is the case then a dressing will be required that will either: debride the chronic granulation tissue and kick-start the process; or restimulate activity in the granulation tissue bed.
- Is the wound static? Wounds which are not healing or where wound healing appears to have stopped need to be investigated fully; this may mean taking a biopsy to check for neoplasia, e.g. presence of mast cell tumours, and assessing the systemic condition of the animal, e.g. underlying diseases such as hyperadrenocorticism, diabetes mellitus. Is there the presence of other tissue which may be inhibiting healing, e.g. exposed bone.

The condition under which the wound was created also needs to be taken into consideration as this will affect how much intervention is required. A clean laceration less than 6 hours old will require less preparation than a dirty shearing injury involving a joint. There are no wound dressings which can compensate for the inadequate cleaning, preparation and debridement of a wound, treatment of other injuries or provision of analgesia.

As previously mentioned, during the treatment, wounds need to be closely observed so that the changes in the wound as it heals are noted to ensure the most appropriate dressing is chosen and used as healing progresses. It is most important to ensure the dressing changes are made at appropriate intervals to optimise the healing process. During the initial stages of the wounds' treatment it may be easier and more effective to hospitalise the patient to allow the dressing changes to be made as frequently as is required and also to ensure the dressings do not become contaminated during the critical early healing phases. There is nothing more frustrating than to see a wound healing well and to discharge the patient with specific dressing care instructions to the owner, only to see the patient return 48 hours later with the dressing contaminated with 48 hours' worth of urine and a wound which is now infected with areas of necrosis.

IDEAL CHARACTERISTICS OF DRESSINGS

These include:
- Non-toxic
- Non-irritant
- Non-allergenic
- Absorbent
- Sterile
- Cost effective
- Allowing gaseous exchange of oxygen and carbon dioxide
- Vapour permeable
- Providing thermal insulation
- Maintaining a moist environment
- Promoting wound healing.

PASSIVE DRESSINGS

ADHERENT DRESSINGS

The primary function of adherent dressings is to debride necrotic tissue from wounds and to control infection within contaminated wounds. Their use is generally indicated during the early stages of wound healing (debridement stage) where some debridement of the wound is required. The decision at this stage is between the placement of a wet or dry dressing, and this will be determined by the amount of exudate/transudate from the wound.

Dressings adhere to wounds by one of two processes:

- Proteinaceous exudate penetrates the dressing, which then dries out as the exudate is absorbed into the secondary (absorbent) layer

or

- There is penetration of the dressing mesh by granulation tissue; this process however indicates that a dressing has been left in place for too long.

Table 4.1 Advantages and disadvantages of adherent dressings

Advantages	Disadvantages
Excellent debridement	Painful to remove
Good at combating infections, especially Pseudomonas infections	Damage surrounding healthy tissue and can macerate surrounding skin if too wet
Cheap	Must be changed frequently
	Damage healthy wound bed

The most commonly used adherent dressings within small animal practice are probably 'wet-to-dry' or 'dry-to-dry' dressings. These dressings consist of mesh cotton gauze, i.e. sterile surgical gauze swabs. These types of dressings are used to aggressively debride infected or necrotic wounds or occasionally for wounds with excessive granulation tissue or to restimulate the granulation bed in a static wound.

Wet-to-dry dressings

These dressings are created by wetting sterile gauze dressings in sterile Hartmann's solution or 0.9% sodium chloride solution. The dressing is then squeezed out until the majority of the fluid has been removed or a limited amount of fluid is applied to the swab, and the dressing is then applied to the wound, ensuring it conforms well to the wound surface. There needs to be very little moisture remaining in the swab before it is placed on the wound or the gauze will not adhere to the wound and perform its function. This dressing must then be covered with a highly absorbent secondary layer followed by a tertiary layer to hold the layers in place. The fluid within the gauze then dilutes any exudate produced within the wound and this exudate then soaks into the gauze which then dries out, allowing necrotic material, pus and debris to adhere to the gauze dressing. This material is then hopefully removed when the dressing is removed (Fig. 4.1). Again, if too much moisture is left within the swab then the necrotic material will not adhere to the dressing and the results will be disappointing, resulting in further dressing placement, although this is largely dependent upon the level of exudate produced by the wound. The purpose of this dressing is to debride the wound and therefore it must be changed at least once every 24 hours or more frequently if large amounts of exudate are being produced or large amounts of debris or necrotic tissue require removal. Care needs to be taken when applying the dressing as, if it is too wet when applied, bacterial strikethrough and tissue maceration may occur. In addition, the secondary layer may not have the capacity to absorb such large volumes of fluid and hence the dressing will have been useless as it will not have adhered to the wound surface. Good quality swabs should always be used as inferior quality swabs will leave lint behind in the wound bed.

These dressings are very useful in patients with shearing injuries, following road traffic accidents, particularly where large amounts of debris, e.g. gravel, organic matter, is embedded within the wound. Wet-to-dry dressings may be placed following initial lavage and cleaning of the wound, to be removed 12–24 hours later to allow surgical debridement or reconstruction to take place. The decision may also be taken to place further wet-to-dry dressings in order to mechanically debride the wound further if the surgeon is hesitant about removing excess amounts of tissue. Care also needs to be taken with the placement of such dressings over vital structures, e.g. exposed nerves, arteries, etc.

Dry-to-dry dressings

These dressings are generally used on wounds with large amounts of exudate, foreign matter or necrotic tissue which cannot be removed via surgical debridement.

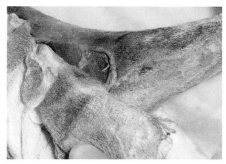

Figure 4.1   Removal of a wet-to-dry dressing

These dressings, as the name suggests, are applied dry to the wound, therefore the dressing has a good absorptive capacity, and debris and necrotic material will adhere well to the dressing. This dressing is again generally left in place for 24 hours so both the contact and secondary layers will have absorbed the exudate and the primary gauze layer will have dried out and adhered well to the wound. The removal of this dressing results in the debridement of the wound. These dressings should be left in place for no longer than 24 hours; if the dressing is left in place any longer then capillary ingrowth may occur and granulation tissue may infiltrate between the mesh of the gauze, which may set wound healing back by several hours or days.

The major disadvantage of both these dressings is that they are very painful to remove and therefore analgesia combined with either deep sedation or general anaesthesia will frequently be necessary to allow removal, which obviously drastically increases the cost of applying such dressings. If dressings are left in place too long, tissue damage may occur on removal, inhibiting wound healing and increasing healing times.

LOW OR NON-ADHERENT DRESSINGS

These types of dressings are used to protect the wound from the environment and bandaging materials. They are useful as, once granulation tissue begins to form, but before the epithelialisation phase, the primary dressing should ideally not be allowed to adhere to the wound, but should have the ability to absorb exudate.

The types of products available vary greatly in their level of adherence, from non-adherent dressings such as silicone mesh dressings used following skin grafting, to the low adherence perforated polyurethane dressings used commonly in practice to cover surgical wounds closed primarily.

Perforated polyurethane membranes

These dressings consist of a thin perforated polyurethane or tetrathiolate (Melolin™) layer, which is coated with an absorbent backing layer, e.g. Melolin™ (Smith &

Table 4.2 Advantages and disadvantages of low or non-adherent dressings

Advantages	Disadvantages
Most are cheap and simple to use	Only the more expensive dressings are truly non-adherent
Do not interfere with normal healing	Do not maintain a moist environment
Some absorb a small amount of exudate	Open wounds will dry out

Nephew). These dressings should be described as low adherence when compared to wet- or dry-to-dry dressings, but strictly speaking are not non-adherent. As these dressings are permeable they will allow wounds to dry out and therefore their use should be restricted to the protection of an elective surgical wound from contamination and trauma and some of these products, e.g. Primapore™ and Meopore™, have adhesive edges making them ideal for this purpose (Fig. 4.2). These dressings, if applied to open wounds, have the disadvantage of adhering to the wound if the exudate is allowed to dry out. Another disadvantage is that the polyurethane layer has small holes which allow gas permeability but it has been demonstrated that capillary loops can grow into these holes, or blood clots may establish fibrin mesh through them therefore making some areas of these dressings adherent; this will result in damage to the tissues upon removal of the dressing, as well as pain for the patient.

One of the mistakes frequently made in practice is the use of such perforated polyurethane membrane dressings in combination with hydrogels, e.g. Intrasite™ (Smith & Nephew). These dressings are often used together to treat granulating wounds as the operator does not fully understand the way in which the various dressings work and how they should be applied. Once such a dressing is applied to a wound, over a period of a few hours the hydrogel begins to dry out and forms a 'crust', which is often partly adhered to both the dressing and the surface of the wound, which in combination with capillary loops adhering to the dressing results in a well adhered dressing which will be particularly painful to remove and will do very little to improve the rate of wound healing. Many veterinary nurses will be familiar with this situation when removing a dressing

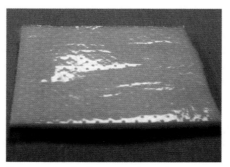

Figure 4.2   Perforated polyurethane membrane dressing

and the resulting pain which it causes for the patient, therefore making further dressing changes more difficult due to the patient's anticipation of the pain.

Paraffin gauzes

These dressings consist of a cotton net or cloth which is impregnated with soft paraffin. The paraffin is present to prevent the mesh from sticking to the wound, but too much of this paraffin can remain within the wound and is frequently difficult to remove without causing trauma to the wound. Excess paraffin may also result in the dressing becoming occlusive by blocking the holes within the mesh, reducing oxygen tension within the wound. Studies have suggested the paraffin inhibits epithelialisation, therefore despite being cheap and readily available these are rarely the dressing of choice.

Silicone mesh

Silicone dressings, e.g. Mepitel™ (tendra), are made from a polyamide net covered with medical grade silicone (Safetac™); this silicone included in the dressing only gently adheres to the stratum corneum, therefore resulting in minimal damage to this layer on removal when compared with other traditional non-adhesive dressings. These dressings are very soft and easy to apply and handle as they are tacky, therefore they stick to intact dry skin but not to moist skin, i.e. the wound itself. As the exudate can pass through silicone mesh, this type of dressing requires a secondary absorptive layer which can be changed easily but without disturbing the underlying dressing itself. These dressings are marketed as single use only but it is possible for them to be washed, autoclaved and re-used once (for use on the same patient) which is advantageous as they are very expensive. These dressings are ideal for use on free skin grafts to prevent the adherence of the primary dressing to the graft.

Vapour permeable films

Vapour permeable films such as Opsite Flexigrid™, IV 3000™ (Smith & Nephew) and Tegaderm™, aid moist wound healing whilst providing a barrier to protect the wound from environmental contamination and trauma. These dressings consist of a thin conformable adhesive film, and they are applied by stretching them over the wound and sticking the dressing to the dry normal skin edges. These dressings are only suitable for low exudate wounds, as the wound exudate becomes trapped beneath the membrane. These dressings have the advantage of creating a moist wound environment whilst at the same time allowing vapour exchange at the wound surface; however they are only suitable for very shallow, non-infected wounds. These dressings are very useful for protecting skin and have been used successfully to cover lick granulomas, prevent pressure sores and as surgical incise drapes. I have used these dressings with great success to cover local anaesthetic creams, whilst allowing them to take effect before obtaining blood samples, collecting blood from donor patients and placing intravenous catheters in fractious patients, especially for rabbit lateral ear vein catheterisation. They are also useful for securing intravenous catheters in place, the purpose for which IV 3000™ dressings were designed, as they are sterile, adhere well if placed correctly and allow visualisation of the catheter/skin interface without removing dressings of tape, therefore allowing for the detection of infection, swelling, etc. These dressings are also very useful for patients who have undergone surgery which may result in urinary incontinence or a recumbent patient and the veterinary surgeon is reluctant to place a urinary catheter. This dressing will help prevent the contamination of the incision site with urine, which may result in an infected wound. These dressings can be tricky to apply and for surgical draping require two pairs of hands and an immobile patient. They are generally only suitable for application to clipped or hairless skin, as they were created for the human market, but their adherence can be enhanced by using alcohol wipes (Skin Prep™, Smith & Nephew) created to degrease the skin prior to application, which also leave a sticky residue, helping to hold the dressing in place. The application of warm hands prior to the removal of the plastic backing layer also appears to improve the adherence. Removal of these dressings can be difficult as, if they have been carefully applied, they may be very well adhered to the patient's skin, and this problem may be overcome with the careful application of small amounts of surgical spirit which will remove the adhesive (see Fig. 4.3).

As previously mentioned, vapour permeable films are also marketed as adhesive surgical drapes. Again, these dressings have the advantage of providing some protection from environmental contamination as well as giving the surgeon the reassurance that the drape will remain secure. Some adhesive surgical drapes have the added advantage of the inclusion of an antimicrobial agent (iodine) within the adhesive itself, e.g. Ioban™ (3M), thus giving improved protection of the wound from environmental contamination by bacteria, therefore reducing the bacterial load of the wound.

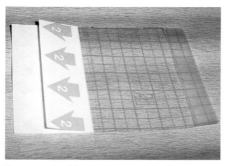

Figure 4.3   Vapour permeable film dressing

ABSORBENT DRESSINGS

The functions of absorbent dressings include:

■ The absorption of fluid exudate from the wound
■ Protection of the wound from the environment
■ Provision of the optimum moist environment for wound healing.

Foam dressings

Foam dressings are a fairly recent development in wound dressings; they were created in order to dress wounds where perforated film type dressings were un-suitable and to overcome the problems they posed for granulating wounds. The primary function of foam dressings is the absorption of fluid, although they also provide a protective barrier over the wound and assist in moist wound healing. Foam dressings are highly versatile and are currently available in many different shapes and sizes. They are available either as flat sheets, for use on superficial open wounds, or as foam chips in a polyurethane bag, for use in wounds with a cavity, e.g. deep ulcers. In small animal practice the flat sheet foam dressings are more commonly used. One of the more commonly used multi-layered dressings (Allevyn™, Smith & Nephew) consists of a perforated non-adherent poly-urethane film, a polyurethane foam, hydrophilic core and an outer polyurethane film (Fig. 4.4).

These dressings have excellent absorptive capacity; they can absorb 10 times their own weight in exudate, and aid wound healing by providing a warm, moist, well oxygenated environment. The backing layer of the dressing allows con-trolled evaporation and acts as an effective bacterial barrier. The foam and backing layer prevents dehydration within the wound and hence minimises any risk of adherence.

Although foam dressings have no bioactivity, such dressings are extremely absorbent, hence maintaining a warm (35°C) moist wound environment which is optimal for granulation and epithelialisation. The creation of the moist wound environment is assisted by the addition of an outer surface which usually consists of a semi-permeable membrane, hence allowing controlled vapour permeability. However, if the wound is not producing sufficient amounts of exudate it will eventually dry out as the moist environment will not be present.

The semi-permeable outer membrane prevents the strike-through of exudate; these factors mean that the dressing will not require changing as frequently as standard dressings with secondary absorbent layers.

Figure 4.5 illustrates the discolouration that may be seen on the backing layer of foam dressings; the secondary and tertiary layers may be removed to allow inspection of the dressing for the extent of exudate absorbtion, without dis-turbing the dressing and therefore the healing wound at all. Hence, if the wound is producing lower levels of exudate then it may remain in situ for up to 5 days.

Nappies and sanitary towels

Nappies and sanitary towels are the ultimate fluid absorbers. They are useful as they can be weighed pre- and post-dressing change to allow an estimation of the amount of fluid which has been lost. In wounds with copious amounts of fluid loss, e.g. open peritoneal drainage, this is a very important part of patient management. In such cases even if the nappies used are non-sterile there may be so much one-way movement of fluid, i.e. out of the patient, that the risk of bacterial migration back into the patient will be minimal.

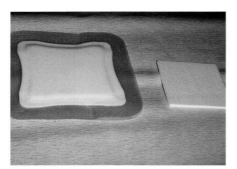

Figure 4.4   Foam dressing (allevyn adhesive (left) and allevyn lite (right))

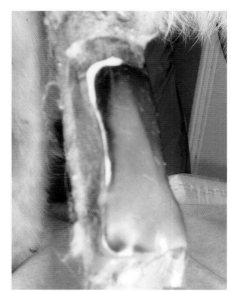

Figure 4.5   Foam dressing in situ

ACTIVE DRESSINGS

These dressings interact with the wound and increase the rate at which wound healing occurs. Moist wound healing is encouraged by the retention of fluid within the wound and debridement of the wound is achieved by rehydration of necrotic tissue, which is then more easily removed by lavage.

HYDROCOLLOIDS

Hydrocolloid dressings, e.g. Granuflex™ (ConvaTec), Tegasorb™ (3M Health Care), are composed of a microgranular suspension of natural or synthetic polymers, including gelatin, pectin and carboxymethylcellulose, in an adhesive polymer matrix. The outer layer of the dressing is usually a semi-permeable film which is shower-/waterproof. In the initial stages these dressings are totally impervious to water and are therefore extremely valuable in rehydrating a wound. As the gel forms, the dressing becomes more water permeable and therefore allows fluid to escape from the dressing; this feature allows hydrocolloid dressings to cope with moderate amounts of wound exudate although they are unable to cope with large volumes. These dressings allow moist wound healing, provide gentle debridement and encourage granulation tissue to form. The bioactivity of these dressings is provided by the release of minute quantities (10–6M) of hydrogen peroxide which has an antioxidant activity in the wound bed, therefore maintaining the reduction potential for cell proliferation and metabolism; this also acts to stimulate an inflammatory response.

The majority of these dressings are waterproof and therefore do not require a secondary dressing if the edges have adhered adequately. The manufacturers of these dressings suggest they may be left in place for up to 7 days, and the wound can be viewed through the transparent outer covering. These dressings, however, should not be used in the presence of infection; therefore they are unsuitable for early debridement of wounds. Breakdown products from the dressing may remain within the wound and if this occurs they have to be removed using lavage at each dressing change. Occasionally this material can be difficult to remove from the granulating wound bed, and the adhesive may irritate the patient's skin. These dressings are most useful in light to medium exuding wounds and have been used successfully to draw out splinters.

HYDROGELS

Hydrogels function by: aiding moist wound healing; providing gentle debridement and encouraging the growth of granulation tissue.

Hydrogels are inert cross-linked polymers with 95% water content and a huge capacity for fluid absorption. The gel swells three-dimensionally and therefore does not put pressure on the wound bed. The most commonly used hydrogels are those in tubes (e.g. Intrasite™, Smith & Nephew), which are applied directly into the wound but they are also marketed as sheet hydrogels with a semi-permeable backing (e.g. Hydrosorb™, Hartmann). The gels must be covered with another primary dressing, therefore increasing the cost of application. The second primary layer used should be a vapour-permeable film, e.g. Opsite, or a foam dressing with a vapour-permeable backing, e.g. Allevyn™; this use of 'double dressings' will increase the cost of dressing the wound, making it quite expensive. These gels should not be applied under a permeable dressing, e.g. Melolin™, as this will allow the hydrogel to dry out, forming crusts within the wound, and making the dressing difficult and painful to remove.

These dressings are useful for dry, sloughing or necrotic wounds, lightly exuding wounds and granulating wounds. The wound is debrided by rehydration of the necrotic tissue, which is much easier to lavage out of the wound bed than hydrocolloid. The debriding activity is achieved without traumatic removal of tissue and hydrogels are much less painful to apply and remove than adherent dressings. The high water absorbence will also reduce oedema and swelling associated with a wound. It has been noted that hydrogels may provide some analgesia to the wound, particularly if the tubes have been stored in the refrigerator for some time before application; it is thought that the molecules rehydrate the wound endings which therefore gives some pain relief.

ALGINATES

These dressings function to: aid moist wound healing and encourage the growth of granulation tissue. The dressings, e.g. Algisite M™ (Smith & Nephew), Kaltostat™ (ConvaTec) are derived from seaweed (giant kelp) and contain varying proportions of guluronic and mannuronic acids. Alginates rich in guluronic acids form solid gels which can be removed from the wound intact, whereas alginates rich in mannuronic acids form soft gels which are removed by lavage. The high sodium content of the wound exudate displaces calcium from the alginate dressing. Calcium stimulates the degranulation of mast cells and the release of pre-formed growth factors into the wound. This may re-stimulate chronic granulation tissue, or encourage the formation of new granulation tissues in areas where it normally develops slowly, in previously irradiated sites, indolent wounds or bony surfaces.

Although these dressings cannot debride necrotic tissue, they can be used safely where there is evidence of infection. Alginates were originally developed as haemostatic dressings (as the clotting cascade is stimulated by the release of calcium ions). Moist wound healing is achieved by gel formation but the majority of veterinary alginate dressings require a secondary dressing on top. Alginate dressings require moistening with saline on application or activation by absorption of wound fluid; the dressings should always be trimmed to the shape of the wound as dry fibres will irritate the patient's skin. Alginate dressings should not be placed in deep wounds or within body cavities as they can initiate a foreign body reaction, as they are not designed as absorbable haemostatic agents for intraoperative use.

Alginate dressings generally require changing every 2–3 days (see Fig. 4.6).

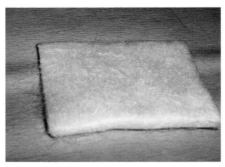

Figure 4.6   Alginate dressing

COLLAGENS

The function of collagen dressings is to promote the growth of granulation tissue and epithethelialisation. The past few years have seen an expansion in the use and range of collagen products in the veterinary market, with collagens such as Collamend™ (Genitrix), Biosist™ (Arnolds) and Emovet™ (Nelson Veterinary) widely available. The products, although differing in their composition, are all essentially sheets of collagen or lyophilised tissue with a high collagen content. The collagen may reduce wound contraction and improve the deposition of organised matrices of collagen fibres. It is thought that earlier deposition of organised granulation tissue may allow earlier epithelialisation as the cells have a matrix across which they can travel. Wound contraction, however, despite not being of benefit in human medicine, is a great contributor in veterinary patients, contributing 30% to wound closure. Some consideration should be made to the use of these dressings in infected wounds as the bacteria will use the collagen as a food source, which will ultimately assist bacterial replication and therefore result in further contamination of the wound, although there is no scientific evidence to substantiate this.

TOPICAL PRODUCTS

BARRIER FILMS

Barrier films, e.g. 3M™ Cavilon™ No Sting Barrier Spray (3M Health Care, see Fig. 4.7), OpSite™ spray (Smith & Nephew), are used to protect intact skin from from bodily fluids, adhesives, friction, scald or pressure. The films are non-sting, transparent sprays or foams which dry onto intact skin and create a water-proof barrier. These products are highly effective, protecting the skin from irritation and scald associated with saliva, urine, sweat, faeces, etc. and are highly useful in the nursing of recumbent patients.

The uses of barrier spays are endless but they are particularly useful for:

- Application to the perineal region of patients following pelvic trauma or surgery where patients are suffering from urinary incontinence
- Application to lip fold of patients with lip fold dermatitis following cleaning with chlorhexidine gluconate solution and thorough drying
- Application to the mouth area of cats following head trauma and mandibular fracture where excessive salivation is a problem
- Application to perineal region of patients with diarrhoea
- Application to the patient's skin to prevent clipper rash
- Protection of the skin from the eczema associated with Elizabethan collars and prolonged bandaging
- Protection of the patient's skin from irritation when adhesive or tapes are used to hold dressings or cannulas in place.

The spray dressing can be topped up every 48 to 72 hours; there is no need to remove the film from the skin as it will naturally peel off.

CLEANSING SOLUTIONS

Cleansing agents, e.g. Aserbine™ (Goldshield) and Dermisol™ (GlaxoSmithKline), are marketed as either a solution or a cream, composed of malic, benzoic and salicylic acid in propylene glycol. These are debriding agents which can be used to cleanse wounds; they act by causing separation between dead and living tissue. They have a very low pH, 2.4, and can irritate the surrounding normal skin. Their action as debriding agents means they are toxic to healthy granulation tissue and therefore should only be used on infected or necrotic tissue. The solution is approximately six times more concentrated than the cream and should

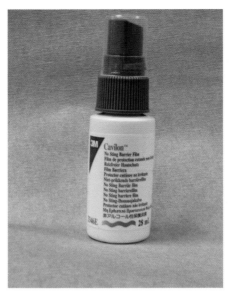

Figure 4.7   3M™ Cavilon™ No Sting
Barrier Spray (reproduced with permission)

always be washed off after application. Neither the solution nor the cream should be left on the wound long term; in addition they are highly unsuitable for the cleansing of inflamed skin or ear canals.

POULTICES

The main constituent of the poultice Animalintex™ (Robinson) is boric acid. The use of boric acid in poultices developed for the human market has long since been banned. The theory behind the use of the poultice is that it will 'draw out' infection or foreign material. This is achieved by vasodilation, oedema and softening of tissues (which include healthy intact skin) and by causing the tissues to produce exudate. These processes are all detrimental to the process of wound healing and the inflammation produced during the process may delay wound healing. Foreign bodies should be removed via surgical exploration and abscesses should be allowed to drain by lancing and lavage under sterile conditions.

ALOE VERA

This product actively promotes wound healing, however only pure forms of aloe vera should be used in wound management.

MAGGOTS

Maggots can be viewed as the ultimate debriding agent. In human wound management larval therapy is becoming increasingly popular as a method of gently debriding wounds. The concept of larval therapy has been around for several hundred years and it was only the introduction of antibiotics in the 1940s that resulted in their decreased popularity. The maggots are effectively the first stage larvae of *Lucilia sericata,* the greenbottle fly. These larvae have underdeveloped mouthparts and feed on liquid protein (i.e. the exudate and necrotic or infected tissue from the wound). Once they develop into second stage larvae, the mouthparts can damage the skin, but they will still only feed on dead cells, exudate, secretions and debris, leaving the live tissue alone. Maggots are suitable for use on superficial wounds and are left in situ for a maximum of 3 days, after which they are removed by flushing out the wound and are replaced with a new batch. Larval therapy is becoming increasingly common in the human field but currently there have been no controlled trials carried out in the veterinary field.

In human wounds, approximately 10 larvae per cm^2 are introduced into the wound and held in place by a piece of sterile net. This net is then attached to a hydrocolloid dressing and secured with adhesive tape, in order to prevent the maggots from escaping. The hydrocolloid dressing protects the surrounding skin from the action of the proteolytic enzymes produced by the larvae and stops the larvae from migrating onto intact skin.

This 'dressing' is then left in place for 48–72 hours, after which time the larvae are washed off the wound, and the wound can then be reassessed.

HYDROPHILIC CREAM

Flamazine™ (Smith & Nephew) is a hydrophilic cream containing silver sulphadiazine 1% w/w. The silver sulphadiazine inhibits the growth of virtually all bacteria and fungi in vitro, and is the agent of choice for the prevention of Gram-negative sepsis in human burns patients. Importantly, there is evidence to show that silver sulphadiazine has antibacterial action against methicillin resistant *Staphylococcus aureus* (MRSA), *Pseudomonas* species and enterococci. The antibacterial action is prolonged as the silver ions are gradually released and adhere to the bacterial cell surface, resulting in cell death. Silver sulphadiazine cream should only be applied to the wound as it will cause maceration of the surrounding skin; the wound should then be covered with an absorbent secondary dressing.

This broad spectrum antibacterial property has resulted in the successful use of Flamazine™ in the treatment of pyodermas and other similar bacterial related skin problems.

SILVER DRESSINGS

More recently, a new silver dressing has been produced; an antimicrobial barrier dressing with Nanocrystalline silver (Acticoat™ with SILCRYST™ Nanocrystals). This product contains nanocrystalline silver. The silver is present as minute silver Nanocrystals (average size 15 nm), which are arranged in a loose, coarse columnar structure in order to provide a large surface area so as to encourage the continuous release of silver ions into the wound.

The metallic silver present in the Acticoat™ dressing is relatively inert, but when moistened with exudates from wounds, the interaction which takes place between the fluids results in the release of silver ions. The dressing acts when the silver ions bind to and denature bacterial DNA and RNA and hence inhibit bacterial replication.

The silver molecules become bound within the wound; this silver continues to have antibacterial activity long after the wound exudate has resolved. It has been demonstrated that the bacteria and yeasts present in wounds take up and concentrate silver from even very dilute solutions. This dressing actively encourages the formation of granulation tissue. This nanocrystalline silver coating has several unique functions: it provides an antimicrobial barrier, it allows the rapid sustained release of silver ions (70–100 ppm) into the dressing and to the wound bed for up to 3 days (Acticoat™) or 7 days (Acticoat™ 7). The dressing aids wound bed preparation by effectively reducing the bacterial load in wounds and prevents and reduces colonisation and infection by killing wound bacteria, and therefore results in increased healing rates. It demonstrates rapid bacterial kill rates, which includes MRSA and VRE, in as little as 30 minutes, showing effectiveness against more than 150 wound pathogens. The killing of several strains of odour-causing bacteria results in reduced wound odour.

Acticoat demonstrates a very broad spectrum of activity, inhibiting more than 150 organisms. In addition, the nanosilver product has been shown to be as effective against yeasts and common fungal pathogens (see Fig. 4.8).

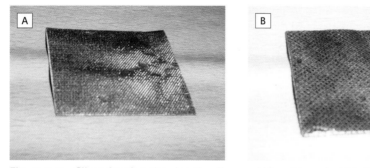

Figure 4.8   Silver dressing showing the silver and blue sides, of which the blue side should always be placed next to the wound

SUGAR PASTE AND MANUKA HONEY

Both sugar paste and honey have been used for centuries to treat wounds; they were reportedly an effective topical wound agent used by the Egyptians around 1600 BC. Sugar pastes have been developed for clinical use by combining caster sugar and additive free icing sugar dissolved in hydrogen peroxide and polyethylene glycol 400. The theory is that the sugar paste lowers the pH of the wound to approximately 5, and helps to debride infected or dirty wounds. The sugar competes with bacteria for water and is therefore antibacterial. The advantage of sugar paste is that it is cheap and readily available. It is not suitable for use on granulating wounds and can be painful on application.

Manuka honey has two positive effects: it is bacteriostatic and it helps with wound cleansing. The bacteriostatic effect is achieved by its low pH (3.7) which is achieved at the wound surface. This low pH has been shown to kill and inhibit streptococci and coagulase-positive staphylococci. The cleansing effect of honey is due to its high osmotic pressure which draws in fluid from the tissues.

Manuka honey for clinical use must be sterile to avoid contamination with clostridial spores and *Bacillus* species and should be derived from pathogen and pesticide free hives. The high osmotic potential assists in the debridement of wounds and helps to draw out exudate from the wound bed. Honey also has an anti-inflammatory effect and promotes the rapid formation of granulation tissue. Excessive exudate will dilute the honey and reduce its osmotic effects, but as honey also contains antibacterial products it will still control infection.

TIME CONCEPT

Over the past decade human medicine has developed a framework for wound management which provides a more structured approach to wound bed preparation and the management of chronic wounds and ultimately aids the clinician in the selection of the most appropriate dressing type for a particular wound in a much more structured fashion.

These wound bed preparation principles have been summarised in the 'TIME' concept. This concept has been modified to make it much more 'user friendly' by the European Board of Wound Management to:

- **T**issue management
- **I**nflammation and infection control
- **M**oisture imbalance
- **E**pithelial advancement.

TISSUE MANAGEMENT

T in the TIME framework analyses the relationship between a wound's appearance and its pathophysiology. An improved understanding of the relationship between the wound's appearance and its pathophysiology and all the underlying cellular and biochemical events which are occurring within the wound allows us to make a knowledge based decision in order to assist the wound healing process.

If faced with a chronic wound which is not healing as expected, then appropriate intervention and treatment will be required to convert a wound from one which is non-healing into a healing state. In order to do this by the route which will be fastest, and will produce the best outcome from a cosmetic and functional viewpoint, a detailed assessment of the wound will be required.

Table 4.3 Types and uses of dressings

Dressing type	Indications	Aims/action
Adherent dressings Dry-to-dry dressings	Copious, low viscosity exudate – infected or necrotic, inflammatory healing phase	Debridement of the wound surface at each dressing change
Wet-to-dry dressings	Low exudate, but high viscosity – infected or necrotic, or chronic granulation tissue	
Non-adherent dressings **Semi-occlusive** Perforated film dressings	Granulating wound	Protection of the wound surface: allows epithelialisation and absorption of exudate
Paraffin gauze dressings	Granulating wound, early repair phase	As above: allows more exudate through into the secondary layer. Paraffin may inhibit epithelialisation. Increases wound contraction
Kaltostat – calcium alginate	Granulating wound, heavy exudate Moisten with saline and trim to fit the shape of the wound	Stimulation of macrophage debridement whilst allowing haemostasis, epithelialisation and absorption of exudate. Pad forms a gel when absorbing exudate, which cleans the wound
Occlusive (Non-adherent) Hydrocolloids	Healthy granulating wound. Contraindicated in the presence of infection or incomplete debridement Exudate remains trapped on the wound surface and may encourage bacterial proliferation	Provide a moist environment for the proliferative phase of healing, i.e. once granulation tissue is established, and encourages rapid epithelialisation
Foam dressings	Exuding wounds during inflammatory phase or wounds during repair phase with granulation tissue and minimal exudate; useful for covering hydrogels	Absorb fluid and increase epithelialisation by creating moist wound environment, may result in tissue maceration and bacterial proliferation

table continues

Dressing type	Indications	Aims/action
Hydrogels	Use in dry, necrotic or sloughing wounds, in combination with foam dressings	Maintain moist wound environment and permit autolytic debridement
Silver dressings	Heavily contaminated, infected or necrotic wounds generally used in combination with foam dressings	Silver molecules have antibacterial properties by inhibiting bacterial replication. Actively encourage the formation of granulation tissue

- Clinical observations – visual assessment can be used in order to determine the health of the wound bed. This will include the type of tissue, the colour, texture and hydration; all these usual factors can help assess the status of the wound bed. These factors indicate how wound healing is progressing and how effective the treatment so far has been.
- Type of tissue and its colour – observation of the type of tissue present in a wound has always been the most important factor in wound assessment. This includes recording the presence of any necrotic tissue, sloughing, granulation tissue or the presence of epithelialisation.
- We can use this information to assist in the prediction of the wound's state of healing. The various stages of wound healing include: inflammation, reconstruction, proliferation and maturation. The presence of any non-viable tissue within a wound is greatly significant as it may be responsible for delayed healing. Non-viable tissue may be described as necrotic, sloughy, devitalised or dead tissue. Necrotic tissue is normally black or blue and of hard, soft or liquefying consistency. It consists of dead cells and debris, while slough or fibrinous material consists of fibrin, pus and proteinaceous material and is usually creamy yellow in appearance because of the large number of leucocytes present. Interpreting the colour of a wound may cause problems: for example, darker pink granulation tissue may be unhealthy, so other criteria are needed.
- Texture – the surface appearance of a wound can often give other clues so it is important to be able to distinguish between healthy and unhealthy granulation tissue.
- Hydration – how well a wound is hydrated can give the clinician information about moisture levels within the wound. However, it should be remembered that increased wetness may indicate the presence of infection. The amount of wound exudate rapidly decreases in healing acute wounds but high exudates may become a problem in chronic wounds. The composition of the exudate produced also changes as a wound becomes chronic.
- Wound pathophysiology. The appearance of a non-healing wound is the outcome of the interaction of many cells and their products within the wound environment. Normal healing is characterised by a progression through the

phases of haemostasis, inflammation, granulation and re-epithelialisation. In contrast to this, chronic or indolent wounds re-epithelialise at a delayed rate. There are many reasons why wounds do not progress through the normal healing stages. In order to pinpoint why a wound is failing to heal, it is important to consider the wound's cellular environment as a whole. The healing process in chronic wounds is halted at the inflammation stage. It is when this chronic inflammation is started that the type and quantity of factors which are produced by macrophages change and there is also an increased number of neutrophils found within the wound; these result in the production of large amounts of proteases. This results in the development of chronic inflammation as there are still persistent inflammatory stimuli within the wound. One such highly relevant and potent stimulus is bacteria, whose presence within a chronic wound are considered to be a contributing factor to the development of the wound. Inflammation itself is a response to tissue trauma or damage, and the products of proteolytic tissue degradation with the accumulation of necrotic tissue will also result in the stimulation of chronic inflammation. Culture of almost all chronic wounds will result in a positive result for bacteria and this problem needs to be controlled before wound healing can progress.

INFECTION CONTROL

Chronic wounds frequently contain high loads of bacteria or fungi. This is partly due to chronic wounds remaining open for longer periods, but also due to the poor blood supply, hypoxia and underlying disease processes. The incidence of infected wounds is associated with prolonged wound healing times which results in greater stress for the patient as a result of repeated dressing times, general anaesthetics and antibiotic administration, as well as increased costs and time for the owner.

In canine patients, the infections of wounds are usually associated with *Staphylococcus* spp., although *Escherichia coli* and anaerobic bacteria, such as *Bacteroides,* with *Clostridium,* often contaminate wounds located near the rectum.

In cats, *Pasteurella* is a commonly isolated bacterium from soft tissue infections, particularly cat bite abscesses.

Organisms grow synergistically: for example, aerobic organisms consume oxygen, leaving tissues devoid of oxygen, hence favouring the growth of anaerobes. Other mechanisms include: producing nutrients for use by other bacteria or impairing the host's immune system.

The assessment and diagnosis of infected wounds can be difficult as chronic wounds do not always display classic signs of infection and hence other criteria must be taken into account.

Another factor which should also be considered is that in human patients the signs and symptoms of infection may be absent or reduced in patients with diabetes and the use of immunosuppressive drugs may mask the signs of localised or systemic sepsis. It has more recently been revealed that when bacteria multiply they form micro-colonies that become attached to the wound bed and secrete a glycocalyx known as 'biofilm' that helps to protect the microorganism from anti-microbial agents which, in turn, may result in delayed healing.

Diagnosis of infection

Obtaining a good history plays a vital role in determining the age and nature of a wound. Observations provide a clinical diagnosis which can be supplemented with microbiological data.

Swab or biopsy?

Wound biopsy, allowing quantification of bacteria, has been considered the gold standard. However, in reality, the cost of surface sampling, i.e. swab for culture, is significantly less and can be performed during a consultation without sedation or general anaesthesia. Both the type and quantity of bacteria present are important, as some bacteria cause injury with a much lower dose than others. The standard cotton wool swab is used generally in first opinion practice and this gives a good indication as to the presence of bacteria within wounds so that careful antibiosis can be selected.

Patient assessment

The patient should be assessed as a whole to identify those who are more likely to develop infection. Factors considered likely to increase the chance of infection are:

- reduced tissue perfusion
- metabolic disorders such as diabetes
- corticosteroids
- large wound area
- chronicity of the wound
- necrotic tissue
- foreign bodies.

Wherever possible, these factors should be removed.

The wound assessment should be recorded, including the measurements of the wound, and where possible, photographic evidence of the size of the wound. This provides a reliable comparison for a later date.

Reducing the bacterial load of a wound

There are a number of ways to reduce the bacterial burden:

- enhancing host defence mechanisms
- wound debridement; where the presence of necrotic tissue in the wound bed is associated with wound infection, and debridement reduces the risk of infection; it also enhances the host's defence mechanism by reducing the amount of devascularised tissue

- wound cleansing, where organisms are physically removed by copious lavage using lactated Ringer's solution or saline; the use of gauze swabs should be avoided as they can leave foreign bodies behind
- increased frequency of dressing change; infected wounds often produce large amounts of exudates which may promote bacterial growth, leading to further tissue breakdown
- use of topical antimicrobials.

Antimicrobial strategy

Ideally, topical agents should represent the first line of treatment. In human medicine, sustained release dressing formulas are commonly used; however, in veterinary practice the use of such topical antimicrobial dressings has been limited. Problems which clinicians often face include: the area needs to be closely clipped in order to ensure good contact between the dressing and the patient's skin, the dressing requires protection from interference by the patient, i.e. chewing, licking, scratching, and physical protection from environmental contamination, such as moisture and dirt. However, there are many advantages to using such antimicrobial dressings including:

- they do not interfere with the natural protective bacterial flora found in other parts of the body, i.e. gastrointestinal tract
- they are less likely to induce an allergic reaction.

Topical antimicrobials are not suitable for use on highly infected wounds with soft tissue invasion or systemic sepsis and should not be used as a substitute for debridement.

THE ROLE OF SILVER DRESSINGS IN THE CONTROL OF BACTERIAL RESISTANCE

In human hospitals, and more recently in veterinary practice, there is great concern regarding the emergence of antibiotic resistant bacteria. It is in the prevention and treatment of such antibiotic resistant bacteria that silver antibiotics are thought to play a particularly useful role, as the nanocrystalline silver of Acticoat™ provides a very rapid 'bacterial kill' within 30 minutes.

WOUND SIZE MEASUREMENT

The simplest method of assessing and monitoring wound healing over time is to make and record a sequence of measurements of the size of the wound. However, in veterinary practice this is rarely carried out despite the fact that in human medicine, studies have demonstrated that change in wound size over the first few weeks is an excellent predictor of the future wound healing. The use of routine measurement has another advantage: it allows the early detection of any deterioration in wound healing which may occur as a chronic wound becomes infected. Such a simple early warning system can result in prompt intervention and modification of treatment and hence the re-establishment of wound healing. Human wound measurement is regularly carried out; there appears to be a greater understanding that the early identification of wounds which are not responding as expected to treatment can improve the wounds' outcome and save on time and money. Visitrak™ is a wound measurement device that allows the accurate tracking of a wound's progress. This is a very detailed piece of equipment which digitally calculates the percentage of the wound which is granulating or non-viable, and accurately measures the wound size and depth; it can be used on all types of wounds.

Epithelialisation is the final phase of wound healing; in this way it may be considered the final component in the TIME framework. However, even once the process of epithelialisation is initiated, re-epithelialisation may not always progress onto full wound closure without complications. Continual assessment of wound healing is still required as an integral component of TIME in order to ensure that timely intervention and decision making are successfully implemented.

WOUND BED PREPARATION

One of the first stages in wound bed preparation is to address any client/patient concerns.

Client cooperation is one of the most important factors in the decision making process regarding how to treat a particular wound. The client may have financial or personal circumstances which need to be taken into consideration; hence individual considerations need to be included in the treatment plan.

The concept of wound bed preparation can be viewed as a process of identifying barriers to wound healing, which can be systematically addressed in order to achieve a healthy granulation wound bed that should progress to contraction, maturation and epithelialisation.

Wound bed preparation works well as it provides a systematic and holistic approach to the wound assessment whilst taking individual patients' situations into account. The theory behind wound bed preparation allows the clinician to take a holistic approach to wound management, whilst the TIME framework allows us to focus on the wound bed and healing process itself. TIME allows clinicians to question the processes which are occurring in the wound bed and to present a systematic and scientific approach to wound assessment. TIME also has the additional benefit of assisting less experienced clinicians in their assessment and reassessment of wounds to ensure there are no omissions in the treatment.

Each component of TIME will have an effect on the ability of the wound to move forward in healing, although at different times throughout the healing process, different aspects of the TIME framework will dominate. For example, a necrotic, exudate wound with a high bacterial load may reduce in exudates and bacterial load if debridement of devitalised tissue is performed.

The emphasis here will be on the 'T' (tissue) as that is the greatest barrier to healing at that particular time. Once debridement has been performed there will be a shift in emphasis to the 'I' (inflammatory) aspect, if critical colonisation or local infection continues to be a problem. Once the 'I' has been tackled with the reduction of the bacterial burden of the wound, the wound should then continue to advance towards healing, with a reduction seen in the level of exudates. 'M' (moisture imbalance), which will have been assessed throughout, gives the clinician some idea of the effectiveness of the particular dressing selected, in its ability to maintain the optimal hydration levels to allow the epithelial margin to advance. At this point the 'E' (epithelialisation) becomes the dominant force, while 'M' continues to be monitored.

TIME is a dynamic process which requires regular assessment of the wound in order to achieve optimal wound care. Concentrating on the dominant component of the framework at any given time can be useful when selecting the most appropriate wound dressing.

ADVANTAGES OF TIME

- Using TIME to form an individual treatment plan can provide a baseline of documented information on types of wounds, and dressings and treatment choices.
- Using the TIME framework in a structured way within a practice can highlight specific challenges in areas such as the prevalence of particular wound types which require greater care.
- The ability to determine the change in wound size accurately over time is an extremely useful parameter for differentiating between wounds that are not responding as expected to treatment and those that are progressing well.
- The use of TIME is a dynamic process. It is important to reassess the full TIME framework at regular intervals. TIME highlights the importance of the need to refer back to the previous steps and to consider the perfusion of the wound bed and the possible need for further debridement.

Further reading

Anderson D 2003 Wound dressings unravelled. In Practice 25: 70-83

Baines S 2004 Wound dressings: a review. Veterinary Review 93: 38-42

Mills N, Rolls A 2005 A journey through time: wound bed preparation. Veterinary Times, 4th and 11th Apr 2005

Swaim SF, Henderson RA 1997 Small animal wound management, 2nd edn. Williams and Watkins, Baltimore

Williams JM 1999 Open wound management. In: Manual of canine and feline wound management and reconstruction. BSAVA, Cheltenham, p 937-946

Chapter 5
Wound closure options
Louise O'Dwyer

This chapter will discuss the assessment and treatment of the wound prior to deciding on its further treatment. Wound preparation is an important factor in the treatment of the wound and the techniques used such as lavage and debridement are important in its preparation prior to either closure or open wound management. Options for the closure of wounds include primary closure, delayed primary closure or secondary closure and a section will be devoted to the differences in these closure options and when they should be used.

This chapter will discuss the anatomy of the skin and relate this to wound closure and reconstruction. It will also discuss the principles of reconstruction, wound closure, suture material choice and suture placement.

WOUND CLOSURE OPTIONS

The options for wound closure are:

Primary closure
Delayed primary closure
Secondary closure
Second intention healing.

PRIMARY CLOSURE

This type of closure is generally performed in the closure of clean or clean-contaminated wounds. Wounds which have been created under aseptic conditions may also be closed primarily, unless a large skin deficit makes this physically impossible.

Contaminated wounds pose a different problem: with some of these wounds it may be possible to close them primarily following careful debridement and lavage, however the risk of infection is higher if this technique is used. In this case the placement of a surgical drain should be considered. If the wound is cutaneous and an en bloc debridement technique is selected, then the wound is normally suitable for primary closure.

DELAYED PRIMARY CLOSURE

If the wound is thought to have been created 2 to 5 days ago, then delayed primary closure is generally selected; this allows time for the wound to be dressed with debriding dressings, e.g. wet-to-dry dressings, in order to decrease the incidence of wound infection, when the wound is considered too contaminated to allow closure of the wound or if there is some concern regarding the viability of tissue. This technique may also be used if debridement cannot be performed on initial presentation or is so extensive that stage debridement is deemed necessary, where the technique considered may be secondary closure.

In practice these wounds are generally covered with a dressing either to debride the surface of the wound, e.g. wet-to-dry, or foam type dressings used in combination with hydrogels in order to rehydrate the wound surface and salvage the maximum amount of tissue. If a wound is particularly necrotic or contaminated, the application of calcium alginate dressings or silver dressings may be required. It is only once all the devitalised tissue or contamination, e.g. foreign material, has been removed from the wound that the wound may be considered suitable for closure.

SECONDARY CLOSURE

Secondary closure is performed if primary wound closure is not possible due to the presence of infection or extensive contamination with foreign material. In this case wound closure is performed once granulation tissue is present; some form of reconstruction technique may be required with secondary closure if large tissue deficits are present. This technique is generally selected for wounds which are thought to be 5 to 10 days old.

The technique involves allowing the wound healing process to continue with the use of the appropriate dressing, in order to encourage the presence of granulation tissue. Once this tissue has formed the skin edges are undermined, apposed and closed as by primary closure.

SECOND INTENTION HEALING

This technique involves allowing the wound to heal by the processes of contraction and epithelialisation. It is a method which is generally reserved for dirty wounds where closure by other techniques is not thought to be suitable or wounds where there is a large tissue deficit and the adjacent skin is not sufficient to allow closure either simply or by the use of skin flaps. This technique generally tends to result in the fairly rapid closure of a wound, as wound contraction is successful in small animals due to the presence of abundant, elastic skin.

This technique, although effective, does possess certain disadvantages:

■ Repeated dressing changes and the use of specific dressings can quickly become very expensive; this problem may also be compounded by the fact that general anaesthesia or sedation may be required in addition to medication such as antibiotics and analgesia.

- Healing times may be prolonged in areas where a large deficit is present.
- The final cosmetic result may not be perfect (hairless epithelium).
- There may be stenosis, or impairment of function of orifices may occur with adjacent wounds.
- A reduction in the range of motion of the limb may occur with wounds in close proximity to joints.
- Wound breakdown(s) may occur if fragile epithelium is present over a large area.

CHOICE OF TECHNIQUE FOR WOUND CLOSURE

Various factors must be taken into consideration when deciding which method of wound closure is most suitable:

- The patient's physical status
- Extent of wound contamination
- Extent of damage to soft tissues
- Vascularity of the tissues
- Amount of adjacent tissues available and suitable for closure.

Most commonly, the technique to be used to close a particular wound may be unclear. Obviously, clean incisional wounds are suitable for primary closure, whereas exudative infected wounds should be treated as open wounds and allowed to heal by secondary intention with the option of converting to secondary closure if possible.

As previously mentioned, wounds which are relatively small but contaminated in regions which have large amounts of loose skin adjacent to them, e.g. dog bite wounds to the thoracic or abdominal region, may be closed primarily following en bloc debridement.

Wounds which may be mildly contaminated may be converted to 'clean' wounds following debridement and lavage, which means they may then be closed primarily. Such wounds however, may benefit from the placement of a surgical drain as they frequently have a higher incidence of wound infection; another option to try to reduce infection rates would be to select the delayed primary closure technique.

This demonstrates how there is no single technique which is more suitable for the closure of a wound. Many wounds may be suited to a variety of closure options; therefore every wound should be viewed on an individual basis and an appropriate treatment plan drawn up.

SURGICAL TECHNIQUE

The technical skills of the surgeon are important in reducing the potential for infection. By the close observations of Halstead's principles of atraumatic, aseptic surgery, tissue contamination and injury are minimised. This will result in the preservation of vascularity, tissue oxygenation and enhancement of wound healing. The elimination of dead space will also significantly reduce the infection rate, as

---

Box 5.1   Halstead's principles of surgical technique

Strict aseptic technique
Gentle tissue handling
Sharp anatomic dissection of tissues
Preservation of blood supply
Meticulous haemostasis
Careful approximation of tissue
Obliteration of dead space
Little or no tension across suture lines

---

will the placement of minimal numbers of finest appropriate gauge suture (as previously mentioned). It is important to minimise the length of the surgery as far as possible since for every hour of surgery the infection rate is approximately doubled.

SUTURING AND TENSION SUTURE TECHNIQUES

Closure of a wound should achieve apposition of the wound edges with no tension across the suture line. Wound healing and/or the sutures will fail if there is persistent tension across the surgical wound, as well as causing discomfort and irritation to the patient, which may result in interference and possible removal of the sutures.

The choice of suture material is important in minimising the adverse effects of the sutures on the surgical wound. Selection of the correct size of suture material is also important. For the majority of dogs, size three metric (2/0) or two metric (3/0) is indicated, while for cats and paediatric use, 2 metric (3/0) or 1.5 metric (4/0) is required. With correct appositional suturing there should be no tension on the suture itself and therefore these areas of suture material should be adequate. If closure is dependent on the strength of the suture, then there is too much tension on the wound and it is likely to break down postoperatively.

The commonest fault of suture technique is to place the sutures too tightly. Allowance should be made for postoperative wound swelling which will cause ischemia at the wound edges if the sutures are tight. Ideally, sutures should be placed loosely across the wound edges, apposing them gently without crushing them. This will allow for postoperative wound swelling, which will seal the wound without placing any pressure on the sutures. Sutures should not be placed too close to the wound edge as the pressure of the suture may increase local collagenase activity and cause suture 'cut out'.

A second fault is to place too many sutures. All sutures cause some irritation, resulting in locally delayed wound healing and an increased risk of infection. This is especially true of subcutaneous absorbable sutures. The minimum number of sutures required to close the wound should be used, and the temptation to increase the number of sutures to prevent wound breakdown resisted by improving the surgical plan. If the dead space cannot be closed easily with a few sutures, then a drain should be placed or a pressure dressing should be applied to obliterate this dead space.

Closure of the skin with simple interrupted sutures may be enhanced by the use of an intradermal suture pattern with an absorbable suture material. This stabilises the skin edges in apposition and thereby lessens the tension on the skin sutures, reducing the risk of 'cut out'. The dermis may be apposed with a simple continuous subcuticular suture or with a few simple interrupted sutures with buried knots. The subcuticular sutures are placed superficially enough to appose the epithelial edges, but not so superficially as to cross into the epidermis and cause irritation. Swaged on needles make placement easier and cause less trauma from drag.

Low friction monofilament nylon or polypropylene are ideal suture materials for cutaneous closure, reducing drag and tear in the placing of the sutures, and minimising tissue irritation. High motion areas should be immobilised, or the suture line designed to cross an area where there will be fewer distractive forces: elbow wounds, for example, should be on the lateral side of the elbow, never on the caudal aspect.

TENSION RELIEVING TECHNIQUES

Walking sutures

Walking sutures are absorbable sutures placed in the subcutaneous tissue to distribute the tension of the advancement of undermined skin over a greater area than the wound edge. They are used in situations where there is ample free skin that can be pulled easily forward to cover the wound. The other advantage of this technique is that it allows simultaneous closure of dead space.

The first bite of the suture is placed in the hypodermis and then into the fascia or subcutaneous tissue, not directly beneath the bite in the skin but closer to the centre of the wound. The effect is that when the suture is tied it draws the skin inwards towards the centre. These sutures may result in 'dimples', where the skin is pulled across the underlying subcutis, but these resolve rapidly as healing progresses.

Although often described, 'tension suture' patterns such as mattress sutures, stents or 'near far' pulley sutures are in fact very rarely indicated. Good suture technique and the use of simple flaps result in faster and more reliable healing, with a better cosmetic result.

Relaxing incisions

The idea of creating further incisions in order to close a wound seems contradictory. However, it is really just a way of manipulating loose skin adjacent to a wound, where apposition of the major/primary wound edges is more important than the creation of another smaller fresh wound nearby. For example, wounds that cannot heal by second intention, such as those overlying exposed bone or an

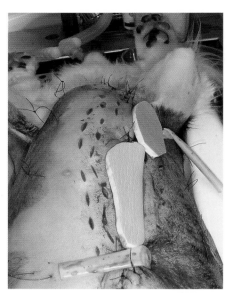

Figure 5.1   The use of relaxing incisions to allow the partial closure of an extensive wound on a patient's chest and abdomen

implant, may be closed, leaving the relaxing incision to heal by contraction, granulation and epithelialisation. The major disadvantage of these techniques is the open wound management of the relaxing incision postoperatively.

Parallel relaxing incisions

A parallel incision is made adjacent to the wound to allow the release of the tension on the suture line (see Fig. 5.1). The skin between the wound and incision is then undermined to allow mobility. The incision should not be so close as to interfere with the original wound. Furthermore, the technique cannot be used on limbs if the skin deficit is greater than 25% of the circumference of the leg.

Multiple relaxing incisions

Alternatively, multiple stab incisions may be used to release tension. This method allows drainage of fluid from beneath undermined areas of skin, and also management of smaller, open wounds (which heal rapidly by second intention). The stab incisions must be staggered to ensure that the blood supply to the skin and wound edges is preserved. This method may be useful for areas where there is movement of the wound site, such as over a limb joint (see Fig. 5.2).

OTHER TECHNIQUES

Most small wounds can be closed if some thought is given to the tension lines, the shape of the wound and the anatomical site. A good general rule is always to

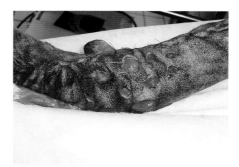

Figure 5.2   Relaxing incisions following the removal of a large mass on a patient's limb to allow the closure of the wound

aim to close the largest area of the deficit first and not give way to the temptation to close the smaller (easier) area first. In this context, planning the excision of a lesion is important, as the shape of the surgical incision can be planned with tension lines and closure patterns in mind. It is always worth, prior to surgery, clipping a much wider area than would appear necessary, allowing adaptation of the surgical plan to allow a flap to be used should it not be possible to close the wound without tension.

MANAGEMENT OF DIFFERENT SHAPES

Depending on their shape, wounds may be approached for closure in various ways. The underlying tension lines of the skin have to be considered – this is done by pushing the skin edges inwards towards the centre of the wound or proposed wound site, and then allowing them to recoil back into place. This gives the surgeon some idea as to how easily the wound edges would come together in a given closure pattern. Wounds should be closed in straight or smoothly curving lines, if possible. However, geometrically shaped wounds can be converted into stellate patterns with straight edges by working inwards from the corners. Occasionally, closure will result in the formation of folds of skin at the edges of a suture line ('dogs' ears' or Burrow's triangles). These should be excised to allow for a more cosmetic result and also to ensure the edge of the suture line lies flat, preventing the formation of fluid pockets in these corners.

Types of wounds have been described in Chapter 2. In practice, wounds which are created electively, under aseptic conditions, e.g. incisional wounds, do not generally create a problem in their closure as they are generally closed in the same direction as they were created. However, elective incisional wounds which have been created following the removal of a large tumour, and consequently the removal of a large area of skin, may be difficult to close correctly, without placing excessive tension on the sutures. Traumatic wounds may also pose similar problems if large skin deficits are present.

SUTURES AND SUTURE SELECTION

SUTURE MATERIALS

Suture materials are classified in many ways in order to describe their characteristics and use within tissues.

Suture materials are classified as absorbable or non-absorbable materials. Absorbable sutures generally undergo degradation and demonstrate a rapid loss in tensile strength within 60 days of implantation, whereas non-absorbable sutures retain a significant amount of strength beyond 60 days. However, this description can be misleading when looking at sutures such as silk, cotton, linen and multifilament nylon, which are all considered non-absorbable but can lose much of their tensile strength within 4 to 6 weeks post-implantation.

Suture material is classified as monofilament (single filament) or multifilament (braided multiple strands). Multifilament sutures are made by twisting or braiding multiple smaller strands of material into a larger suture. Multifilament sutures are generally easier to handle when compared with monofilament sutures. Multifilament sutures also have increased tissue drag due to their irregular surface which can cut through the tissues being sutured. Some multifilament materials are available with a coating to minimise this disadvantage, but this in turn may affect knot security. Monofilament sutures are a single, smooth strand of suture material made by extrusion. These sutures have less tissue drag and decreased bacterial adherence.

The last of the categories for suture material classification is whether the material is natural or synthetic. Natural materials, such as silk, cotton or catgut are generally associated with inflammatory reactions within the tissues and their absorption may be variable depending upon the implant site and patient status. Synthetic materials are usually produced from chemical polymers, and therefore tend to have a much more predictable rate of breakdown and absorption.

The ideal suture material should:

- Be easy to handle
- React minimally within the tissue
- Hold securely when knotted
- Create minimal drag through tissues
- Maintain adequate tensile strength until its purpose is served
- Have rapid resorption once it is no longer required (absorbable)
- Be encapsulated without postoperative complications (non-absorbable)
- Resist shrinkage in tissues
- Be inexpensive
- Be easy to sterilise without changing its material properties
- Not favour bacterial growth
- Be non-capillary
- Be non-allergenic

■ Be non-carcinogenic
■ Absorb with minimal tissue reaction after the tissue has healed.

In reality, such a suture material does not exist, therefore a suture should be selected which most closely matches the ideal properties for the procedure to be performed and the tissue in which it is to be implanted.

SUTURE SELECTION

Suture size

The suture selected should be of the smallest diameter that will adequately hold the tissue whilst healing. This will result in minimal trauma as the suture is passed through the tissue and will also therefore reduce the amount of foreign material within the wound. The suture material and size selected should be no stronger than the tissue to be sutured.

Flexibility

The suture's flexibility is determined by its rotational stiffness and diameter; these properties will influence its handling and its use. Flexible sutures are selected for the ligation of vessels or performing continuous suture patterns. Less flexible sutures (e.g. cerclage wire) is unsuitable for the ligation of small bleeding vessels.

Surface characteristics and coating

The surface characteristics of a suture influence the ease with which it is pulled through the tissues (i.e. the amount of 'drag') and the amount of trauma caused as a result of this 'drag'. Rough sutures may result in more injury to tissues than smooth sutures; therefore smooth sutures play an important role in delicate tissues, e.g. the eye. Smooth sutures, however, require greater tension in order to ensure good apposition of tissues and they have less knot security. Braided materials have increased drag compared to monofilament sutures. To try and reduce this drag, braided sutures are frequently coated in order to provide a smooth surface and to reduce capillarity. Materials used to provide this coating include Teflon™, silicone, wax, paraffin-wax and calcium stearate.

Capillarity

Capillarity is the process by which fluid and bacteria may be carried into multi-filament fibres. Due to the large size of neutrophils and macrophages, they are unable to enter these fibres and as a result infection may persist; this effect is increased in non-absorbable sutures. All braided sutures are capillary, whereas monofilament sutures are less capillary due to their structure. The coating of braided sutures may help to reduce the capillarity of some sutures. The use of capillary sutures is not recommended in contaminated or infected sites.

Knot tensile strength

This is a measure of the force (in kilograms) that a suture strand can withstand before it breaks when knotted. Sutures need to be as strong as the normal tissue through which they are to be placed; however, the tensile strength of the suture should not greatly exceed the tensile strength of the tissue.

Relative knot security

Relative knot security is the holding capacity of a suture expressed as a percentage of its tensile strength. The knot holding capacity of a suture material is defined as the strength required to untie or break a defined knot by loading the part of the suture that forms the loop, whereas the suture material's tensile strength is the strength required to break an untied suture fibre with a force applied in the direction of its length.

General points to consider when selecting a suture

Strength of tissue

A suture should be at least as strong as the tissue through which it passes. A tissue's ability to hold sutures without tearing depends upon its collagen content and the direction in which these collagen fibres run. This helps to explain why ligaments, tendons, fascia and skin are strongest, with muscle being relatively weak (think about abdominal and diaphragmatic ruptures post-road traffic accident), and fat is weakest. Muscle has very little suture holding capability across its fibres and even less in the direction of the fibres. Visceral tissue can be categorised somewhere between fat and muscle in terms of strength.

Use of the smallest suture size possible for wound closure will result in less tissue trauma, allowing smaller sized knots to be tied, and therefore less foreign material to be left within the wound, and forces the surgeon to handle sutures and tissue more carefully. Oversized sutures may weaken the wound through excessive tissue reaction and tissue strangulation.

Healing considerations

The surgeon should consider how the suture will alter the biological processes in a healing wound. Tissues respond to sutures as they would to any other foreign material. The amount of reaction produced is dependent upon the nature of the material implanted (e.g. catgut compared with stainless steel), the amount or surface area of the suture, the type and location of tissue compared with the sutures (intestinal viscera and skin react highly to silk, whereas fascia reacts minimally), the length of implantation and the technique of suture placement (excessive suture tightening results in tissue strangulation). Sutures which result in major tissue reaction are contraindicated in areas in which excessive scar tissue formation may result in functional problems (e.g. for vascular repair or ureteral anastomosis) or cosmetic problems (e.g. in the skin). The surgeon should inflict as little trauma as possible for the operation, reduce contamination and use sutures which will result in the least tissue reaction in order to avoid excess inflammation and delayed wound healing.

All suture materials are capable of increasing wound susceptibility to infection. The chemical and physical structure, capillarity, bio-inertness and ability to adhere to bacteria are all important in suture related infections. Sutures inducing the least foreign body reaction in tissues such as synthetic absorbables and mono-filament non-absorbables produce the lowest incidence of infection in con-taminated wounds.

Wound infection also affects suture integrity. If wound contamination is sus-pected, then synthetic absorbable sutures should be selected as these sutures are more stable and have predictable absorption rates in contaminated tissues. If long-term wound support is required of the suture material, use a synthetic mono-filament non-absorbable or synthetic (prolonged degradation) absorbable suture such as polydioxanone or polyglyconate.

Loss of suture strength and gain of wound strength

To use absorbable sutures safely, the loss of suture strength should be propor-tional to the anticipated gain in wound strength. This factor is important as structures such as fascia, tendons and ligaments heal slowly (50% strength gain in 50 days) and are under constant tensile forces. For these types of tissues, non-absorbable sutures or prolonged degrading, synthetic absorbable sutures are indicated. Monofilament non-absorbable sutures are indicated for skin closure as they induce little foreign body response and the skin has a slower gain in healing strength when compared to visceral healing. General and local factors affecting wound healing must also be considered before an appropriate suture is selected.

Mechanical properties of suture and tissue

The mechanical properties or functions of the suture should be similar to those of the tissue being closed. Less elastic suture materials, such as those composed of polyester fibres, are more suitable for anchoring prosthetic materials or for use in joint surgery.

The surgeon needs to consider these suture principles and select the best suture, on the basis of its physical and chemical characteristics, for the requirements of the tissues being closed. Physical characteristics include durability, handling quality, knot security and heat sterilisation damage. Biological characteristics include mode of absorption, tissue reactivity, predisposition to infection and sinus formation.

In selecting a suture material we need to assess the reason for using the suture. The objective in general is to hold together tissues which have been separated until healing has occurred. Therefore various aspects of suture materials need to be taken into account in making the selection.

SUTURE NEEDLES

There are now almost as many suture needle types as there are suture materials. However, the correct decision on which type of needle to use comes down to four important factors:

How the needle pierces the tissues
The shape of the needle
Attachment of the suture material
Size of the needle.

A needle either pierces the tissues by the use of a cutting edge or a sharp point (taper). Cutting needles have one or more honed cutting edges. These are most useful in strong, dense and organised tissues like skin, fascia, tendons, ligaments and cartilage. There are essentially three types:

- Conventional cutting needles have the inside edge of a curved needle (towards the wound) as the cutting surface.
- Reverse cutting needles have the outside edge of a curved needle (away from the wound) as the cutting surface
- Spatula cutting needles are flattened and are the shape most commonly seen on ophthalmic suture materials.

Taper cutting needles are honed to a fine point at the tip, and are used for less dense tissues, including blood vessels. A taper cut needle tapers to a point, but the point is honed in such a way as to create two or more cutting surfaces. Blunt taper needles have narrow but not sharp points.
    There are essentially three needle shapes:

Straight needles usually have at least one cutting surface, and are almost exclusively used for skin suturing, with some applications for tendon repair.
Half-curved needles are straight in their shaft, but have a curved, cutting tip to them, also used for skin.
Curved needles are formed in an arc of $\frac{1}{4}$, $\frac{3}{8}$, $\frac{1}{2}$, or $\frac{5}{8}$ circle. This allows the surgeon access with the needle to smaller spaces than the straight or half-curved needle, and the arc can be chosen to maximise tissue bite, depth and width.

Suture material can be attached to the needle either by being swaged on or threaded through an eye.

- Eyed needles either have a standard eye that the material is threaded through, or a spring eye in which the eye is split to allow the suture material to be forced into it.
- Swaged needles are pre-drilled and have the material inserted into the base of the needle. This method of attachment is less traumatic as the unit is passed through the tissues. There are also controlled release needles which allow the swaged on suture material to be released from the needle with a firm tug to allow the suture line to be finished with a hand tie.

Needle size is usually divided into heavy gauge, general use and vascular. Vascular needles are designed to be as atraumatic as possible, and to ensure that the size of the needle hole can be completely filled with suture to minimise leakage. Most suture material is supplied with a general use needle with a body thick enough to withstand routine use.

NATURAL SUTURE MATERIALS

These are natural origin sutures which are derived from plant (e.g. cotton) or animal (e.g. catgut, silk) sources.

Absorbable sutures

Surgical gut (catgut)

Surgical gut is made from either sheep intestinal submucosa or cattle intestinal serosa; it has now been taken off the human market by the Medical Devices Agency, but it is still currently marketed for veterinary use (Arnold's sutures). Catgut is a twisted multifilament material whose absorption is very variable, especially in hypoproteinaemic patients, or when used in gastric surgery, an infected wound or highly vascularised tissue. Effective tensile strength for medium chromic catgut is only reported to be 10 to 14 days. In addition, catgut has poor knot security when wet, so the cut end tags should be left longer than would be normal. It can also cause significant foreign body reaction when implanted in tissues.

There are relatively few indications for its use.

Natural non–absorbable sutures

Stainless steel (Steel: USS/DG; Flexon™: USS/DG; Surgical Stainless Steel Suture: Ethicon; Steelex™: Braun)

An alloy made from natural materials, stainless steel is available as a monofilament or braided multifilament suture material (Flexon™). Steel has the highest strength of any other suture material. It is biologically inert and can easily be sterilised by autoclaving. It incites little tissue reaction other than mechanical irritation from the ends. It has excellent knot security, although the knots can sometimes be difficult to place. Pieces of stainless steel can migrate if loose, and it will break if subject to repeated bending. It can easily cut or tear through sutured tissues if tightened too much. Given its difficult handling properties, it is not commonly used in practice as a suture material, but has a wide range of applications in clips and staples. One area, however, where steel suture is still commonly used is closure of sternotomy wounds, as some surgeons feel it gives increased stability compared to PDS II™ or Prolene™.

Silk (Perma-hand™: Ethicon; Sofsilk™: USS/DG; Silkam™: Braun)

Silk has a long history of use as a suture material. It is obtained as a fibre spun from the cocoon of the silk worm, and is available either twisted or braided, but always as a multifilament. Silk has excellent handling characteristics, and is cheap.

However, it has a variety of disadvantages, including some degree of tissue reaction, only marginal knot security and poor tensile strength. Many surgeons prefer the feel of silk, and it is still often used to ligate large vessels, although extended clinical use is limited. It is often moistened in sterile saline before use to improve knot security and reduce tissue drag, although this can slightly decrease its tensile strength. Silk is not recommended in hollow viscera or in infected wounds, as it can potentiate infection by trapping bacteria in its braiding. As with other multifilament materials, use in gallbladder and urinary tract surgery is discouraged as it can be calculogenic.

Cotton

Cotton suture material has similar properties to silk, although it is slightly weaker. It loses half of its initial tensile strength at 6 months, and three-quarters at 2 years. It is also braided and can potentiate infections like silk. It has better knot security, but has electrostatic 'cling' properties that can make it difficult to handle. The tensile strength and knot security are increased when wet. There is also a linen suture with similar qualities manufactured by Braun (Linatrix™). There are no current clinical indications for the use of this material in small animal surgery.

SYNTHETIC SUTURE MATERIALS

Synthetic materials are made from polymers from manmade sources.

Synthetic absorbable sutures – multifilament

Polyglactin 910 (Vicryl ™: Ethicon; Polysorb ™: USS/DG)

This suture material group is composed of glycolic and lactic acids in a ratio of 9:1. This type of material is more hydrophobic (and subsequently more resistant to hydrolysis) than pure polyglycolic acid. These braided materials are coated with a copolymer of calcium stearate to allow less tissue drag and better water-proof properties. It is a relatively strong and easily handled material, with moderately good knot security. Half of the initial tensile strength is lost after 21 days. It incites comparatively little tissue reaction, and is well tolerated in a variety of wound conditions. It is still a braided material, and as such may be liable to wicking of bacteria through the interstices. Polysorb has a smaller braid size than Vicryl™, and although this will not affect the wicking of bacteria, it may give Polysorb™ slightly better knot security.

Lactide/glycoside polymers (Panacryl ™: Ethicon)

Although the material group is similar to polyglactin 910, this has a very different polymer combination. It is a very long-lasting braided absorbable material that absorbs after 1.5 to 2 years. Approximately 80% of the initial tensile strength remains at 12 weeks. Panacryl™ has a coating to minimise drag, and overall the material evokes a minimal tissue reaction. It was originally suggested as an ideal ligament replacement material, as it has improved handling and resists cyclic strain better than monofilament materials. In addition, as an absorbable material, there would be less likelihood of chronic infection. It is currently only available attached to tissue anchors for ligament prosthetics, although it would also be indicated for closure of any tissues that need support for as long as 6 months.

Polyglycolic acid (Dexon II ™: USS/DG; Safi ™l: Braun)

These are also braided suture materials, made from braided polymers of pure glycolic acid. These materials are relatively easy to handle. Absorption is by hydrolysis, although Dexon™ absorption is increased in urine, and so it is not recommended in urinary tract surgery. Polyglycolic acid tolerates infected wounds well, although wicking may be a problem. It is coated to decrease tissue drag and cutting. It is completely gone by 90 days, has better tensile strength than catgut in the critical phases of wound healing, and has approximately 60% strength left at 14 days. Although there may be an initial tissue reaction, this subsides as the wound heals. Knot security is fair, but it will often improve when the material is wet.

Synthetic absorbable sutures – monofilament

Polydioxanone (PDS II ™: Ethicon; MonoPlus ™: Braun)

A polymer material composed of paradioxanone. This is a monofilament with greater strength than monofilament nylon and polypropylene, and with less tissue drag than the multifilament materials. It can sometimes be difficult to handle due to its memory and tendency to coil or 'pig-tail'. Knot security can be relatively poor, and seven throws are advisable at the end of a continuous suture line. Its biggest advantage is a slow and predictable rate of absorption. Only about a quarter of its tensile strength is lost after the first 2 weeks, about half after a month, and most at about 60 days. Absorption is complete by about 180 days, although it does not effectively start until day 90. It incites a minimal amount of tissue reaction. Despite the less than ideal knot security, the strength and predictable rate of absorption makes this an ideal suture material for closure of the abdomen and it has become a very popular material for this use.

Polyglyconates (Maxon ™: USS/DG; Monosyn ™: Braun)

Maxon™ suture material is a polymer of glycolic acid and trimethylene carbonate, while Monosyn™ just contains glyconates. Although slightly stiffer to handle, Maxon™ has a tensile strength and performance similar to polydioxanone, which should be adequate to provide knot security during the critical healing phase of most wounds. Appropriate applications would include, for example, closure of the linea alba. Polyglyconate has been shown to have good knot security. Absorption of Maxon™ starts at day 60 and is completed by macrophages at about 6 months. Monosyn™, on the other hand, has only 50% tensile strength left at 2 weeks, and is gone by 60–90 days. This would be adequate where short-term support is needed, for example subcuticular closure.

Glycomer 631 (Biosyn ™: USS/DG)

This monofilament material is similar to polydioxanone. This is a copolymer of glycolide, dioxanone, and trimethylene carbonate. It is advertised as the strongest monofilament suture material available, second only to steel. A quarter of the strength is gone by day 14, and 40% remains at 3 weeks. The material is gone by day 90 to 110. It has fair handling characteristics with low tissue drag and slightly better knot security than polydioxanone. It is interesting to note that both PDS II™ and Biosyn™ have similar tensile strength for 2 weeks, and although PDS II™ is stronger at 4 weeks, Biosyn™ is absorbed rapidly, which would potentially mean that less material is around once a significant proportion of the tensile strength is lost. This material is promoted as suitable for abdomen closure and soft tissue repair requiring a strong but absorbable suture.

Polyglecaprone 25 (Monocryl ™: Ethicon)

Polyglecaprone 25 is a copolymer of glycoside and epsilon caprolactone. It has very high initial tensile strength and excellent pliability with good knot security. One quarter of its initial strength is gone at 2 weeks, and all at 21 days. It has minimal tissue reaction and rapid absorption. It is a useful material where high initial strength but relatively rapid absorption is required. This material is very useful in subcuticular closure and gastrointestinal surgeries.

Polyglytone 6211 (Caprosyn ™: USS/DG)

This is a synthetic absorbable polyester material indicated for very short-term wound support. Approximately half of its initial tensile strength is gone at day 5, and only 25% remains at day 10. This suture material is completely absorbed by day 56. Interestingly, the absorption rate for this material is the closest of any synthetic material to catgut. Other than perhaps subcuticular closure, there are very few other current clinical indications for the use of this material.

Synthetic non-absorbable sutures

Polyamide/nylon (Ethilon ™: Ethicon; Nurolon ™: Ethicon; Dafilon ™: Braun; Supramid ™: Braun; Dermalon ™: USS/DG; Monosof ™: USS/DG; Surgilon ™: USS/DG)

This family of suture materials is made from amine-containing thermoplastics. Nylon can be found in both braided and monofilament forms. Monosof™, Dermalon™, Dafilon™, and Ethilon™ are perhaps the best known monofilament nylon brands. Supramid™ is classified as a pseudomonofilament – a multi-filament nylon core with a second polyamide nylon cover layer. Surgilon™ and Nurolon™ are both braided nylon suture materials. As a material, nylon is relatively inert, and has no capillary action as a monofilament. Only about 20% of monofilament nylon's initial tensile strength is gone at 1 year, although in some cases all the tensile strength in a multifilament strand can be gone at 6 months. Although monofilament nylon has a reputation for relatively poor handling and knot security, it has a wide range of applications, and is commonly used in a variety of applications including skin, cornea, fascia, and ligatures (e.g. pedicle ligatures for ovariohysterectomy). Due to its stiffness, it is not recommended within hollow viscera, as the cut ends cause mechanical irritation. A minimum of four throws on nylon is always recommended.

In the same family of materials is polymerised caprolactam, a twisted and coated multifilament material with superior initial tensile strength compared to nylon. It has more tissue reactivity than nylon, however: it has been known to cause sinuses when implanted in tissues, so it is best suited for skin. It is generally supplied in bulk rolls, but should not be considered sterile unless processed by ethylene oxide or heat sterilisation. Autoclaving can make it more difficult to handle. In general, this family of materials is best suited for skin sutures. Vetafil™ is a well-known brand of this type of material. Although, in general, multi-filament nylon materials may be easier to handle, the monofilament nylon materials would be preferred for use in the skin because they are less likely to wick outside contaminant bacteria into the deeper tissues of the wound bed.

Polypropylene (Prolene ™: Ethicon; Surgiproll ™: USS/DG; Premilene ™: Braun)

Polypropylene is a widely used synthetic monofilament suture material that is composed of polymerised polypropylene. It is very non-thrombogenic, and is often used in cardiovascular surgery in human patients. It is available as a mesh material for implantation. Polypropylene is very plastic, meaning that the material will assume a new shape when subject to tension, which contributes greatly to its good knot security if the sutures are tightened appropriately. Some surgeons find this material difficult to handle because of its memory and tendency to break if handled roughly. There is no appreciable loss of tensile strength after implantation. The clinical indications for use of polypropylene are varied and include cardiovascular and microvascular surgery, tracheobronchial surgery (e.g. tracheotomies and closure of bronchial stump after lobectomy), gastrointestinal, perineal hernia repair, genitourinary, routine skin closures, and as stay suture material.

Polyester (Surgidac ™: USS/DG; Ti·Cron ™: USS/DG; Mersilene ™: Ethicon; Ethibond Excel ™: Ethicon; Miralene ™: Braun; Dagrofil ™: Braun; Synthofil ™: Braun; PremiCron ™: Braun)

A synthetic, non-absorbable, usually multifilament, suture material that is nor-mally coated, as the suture material has been reported to have some tissue reac-tivity if the coating is lost. Mersilene™ and Miralene™ are monofilament versions. This material has a very high and prolonged tensile strength, although knot security is only moderate. Infection in an area where braided polyester suture has been used almost always necessitates suture removal. Polyester is very strong and has been used most commonly for prosthetic implant placement and large vessel ligations. Given that suture contamination and sinus tract formation with poly-ester materials can be problematic, other suture materials will often provide suffi-cient strength without the risk.

Polybutester (Novafil ™: USS/GD; Vacufil ™: USS/DG)

A special type of polyester material composed of polyglycol terephthalate and polybutylene terephthalate. This makes the material retain many advantages of both polypropylene and polyester. It is delivered as a monofilament, and is commonly used in cardiovascular and ophthalmic procedures. The material is known to have better knot security than polyester alone, with good tensile strength and flexibility.

Polyhexafluoropropylene VDF (Pronova ™: Ethicon)

A special polymer blend of the polypropylene family, this is a relatively new suture material that is designed to be used in cardiovascular and ophthalmic surgery. It has many of the same characteristics as polypropylene and is mainly marketed in similar sizes. Polyester, polybuteser, and polyhexfluoropropylene are not commonly used in small animal surgery.

NUMBER OF KNOTS REQUIRED TO TIE A SECURE KNOT

The number of throws required in order to tie a secure knot is dependent on the suture material and suture pattern.

Simple interrupted pattern

- Stainless steel – two throws (one square knot)
- Polyglactin 910™, polyglycolic acid, surgical gut, polypropylene – three throws
- Polydioxanone, nylon – four throws.

Starting continuous patterns

Add one additional throw for minimum security.

Ending continuous patterns

- Polyglycolic acid, surgical gut, polypropylene – five throws
- Polyglactin 910, nylon – six throws
- Polydioxanone – seven throws.

Interrupted suture patterns

Advantages

- Greater security
- Allow the precise adjustment of tension at each point of suturing.

Disadvantages

- Use more suture material (poor suture economy)

- Leave greater amounts of foreign material (i.e. suture material) within the wound
- More time consuming to place compared with continuous patterns.

STAPLES AND CLIPS

Staples may be used to singly close tissue, such as the skin. Staples are also available in cartridges where all the staples are fired at the same time from a cartridge through the tissues and into an anvil. These staples produce a staggered double row of staples and achieve haemostasis and tissue approximation at the same time. The linear stapler produces one linear double staggered row, the linear cutter produces two linear staggered double rows and cuts between them, and the end-to-end anastomosis stapler produces a concentric circular staggered double row and cuts concentrically.

These staplers are primarily used for partial or complete hepatic and pulmonary lobe resection and gastrointestinal anastomosis. Care should be taken to ensure that the tissue to be stapled is not excessively thick and the staple line should be carefully examined following stapling to ensure that mechanical failure has not occurred.

The advantages of staplers include:

- Speed of use
- Ease of application.

The disadvantages include:

- Cost of staples and instruments
- Necessity to re-sterilise applicators between patients.

TISSUE ADHESIVES (GLUE)

The cyanoacrylates are most widely used. Cyanoacrylate monomers are converted to polymers on contact with water on tissue surfaces. The setting time ranges from 2–60 seconds depending on the thickness of the glue film, the amount of moisture present and the alkyl chain molecules in the glue.

Tissue adhesives have been used effectively in oral surgery, intestinal anastomosis, management of corneal ulceration, control of haemorrhage from the cut surface of parenchymatous organs, microvasculature incisions and skin grafts. Their use in cutaneous wounds and incisions is now widespread.

Problems associated with the use of tissue adhesives include tissue toxicity (with some cyanoacrylates), granuloma formation, potentiation for wound infection, delayed wound healing if edges are separated, poor adherence to moist surfaces and interference with cortical bone healing.

PRINCIPLES OF SUTURE PLACEMENT

- Select the correct size of suture material
- Select the most appropriate material
- Ensure there is no tension across the suture line
- Do not place too many sutures
- Minimise trauma to the skin edges during suture placement.

The most common fault of suture technique is the overtight placement of a suture. It needs to be remembered that there will be some postoperative swelling and if the placement of the suture does not account for this then this will result in ischaemia at the wound edges. Ideally, sutures should be placed loosely across the wound edges, apposing the edges gently without crushing them. This will account for and allow postoperative wound swelling, which will allow the wound to seal without placing any pressure on the sutures. Sutures should also not be placed too closely to the wound edge as the pressure of the suture may result in suture 'cut out'. Sutures should ideally be placed 5 mm from the wound edge and spaced at intervals of 5 mm; this will result in more evenly spread tension along the wound, and minimal interference with local blood supply. If too many sutures are placed, the presence of suture material within the skin always results in some irritation and this may lead to locally delayed wound healing and an increased risk of infection, as well as potentially resulting in trauma to the wound due to patient interference as a result of the discomfort. Ideally, the minimal number of sutures required to close a wound should be used, and the temptation should be resisted to place more sutures in order to prevent wound breakdown; this should be unnecessary if care is taken in the wound closure.

SUTURE REMOVAL

Today non-absorbable sutures are becoming less commonly used in veterinary practice, however there are situations where the placement of non-absorbable skin sutures is necessary. In order to prevent dehiscence, skin sutures should be removed once the skin has healed sufficiently; this is commonly at 10–14 days. However, certain situations require these sutures to remain in place for longer periods of time, e.g. in debilitated animals. Occasionally, the veterinary surgeon may require fibrosis to occur, e.g. in the treatment of aural haematomas, therefore the removal of sutures in such situations may be delayed. Suture removal is commonly performed by a veterinary nurse during postoperative consultations; this task is generally performed with the use of a specifically designed stitch cutter or a pair of suture removal scissors. The ears of the knot are lifted away from the skin, so the blade of the stitch cutter or scissors can be slipped carefully beneath the suture to cut it. Gentle tension on the ear of the knot will result in the suture slipping through the skin and therefore its removal.

SUTURE PATTERNS

Suture patterns may be classified as interrupted or continuous, by the way in which they appose the tissues or by which tissues they primarily appose (e.g. subcutaneous or subcuticular). Appositional sutures (e.g. simple interrupted sutures) bring the tissues in close approximation; everting sutures (e.g. continuous mattress sutures) turn the tissue edges outward, away from the patient and towards the surgeon. Inverting sutures (e.g. Lembert, Connell and Cushing sutures) turn tissue away from the surgeon, or towards the lumen of a hollow viscus organ.

Subcutaneous and subcuticular sutures are placed in order to eliminate dead space and provide some apposition of skin so that less tension is placed on skin sutures.

Subcutaneous sutures tend to be placed in a simple continuous pattern, but in certain situations, e.g. where drainage may be required, a simple interrupted pattern may be more suitable. Subcuticular sutures may be used in place of skin sutures in order to prevent the need for suture removal in a fractious patient or to reduce the incidence of accidental suture removal by the patient. The suture line is started by burying the knot in the dermis. The suture then progresses through the subcuticular tissue, with the bites through the tissue being parallel to the long axis of the incision. The suture line is ended with a buried knot. Absorbable suture material is preferred for subcuticular sutures for obvious reasons.

INTERRUPTED SUTURE PATTERNS
Simple interrupted sutures (Fig. 5.3)

This suture pattern is created by inserting the needle through the tissue on one side of the incision or wound, passing it to the opposite side of the wound and tying the knot. The knot should be created at one side so that it does not directly overlie the incision; the ears of the knot should be left a suitable length to allow them to be grasped during the removal of the sutures. As previously mentioned, the sutures should be placed approximately 3–5 mm away from the skin edge.

This suture pattern will result in good apposition unless excessive tension is placed on the suture, which may result in the inversion of the wound, and the subsequent poor healing of the wound. One of the main advantages of simple interrupted suture patterns is the fact that if one of the sutures should fail this does not result in the failure of the entire suture line. This pattern however, does take more time to place than a continuous suture pattern and will result in more foreign material, in the form of knots, in the wound.

Horizontal mattress sutures (Fig. 5.4)

The horizontal suture pattern is placed by inserting the needle on the far side of the incision, passing it across the incision, and exiting on the far side of the incision, passing it across the incision, and exiting the suture on the near side.

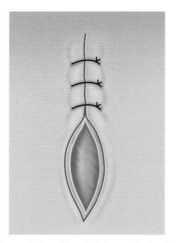
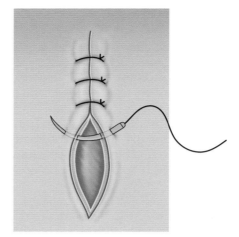

Figure 5.3   Simple interrupted suture pattern

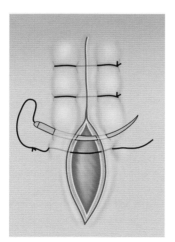
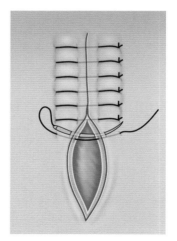

Figure 5.4   Horizontal mattress suture pattern

The needle is then advanced 8–10 mm along the incision and re-introduced, exiting from the skin on the far side, and the knot is tied. This suture pattern is commonly used in areas which are under tension and can be placed fairly quickly; however, they may result in eversion of the wound edges. Care should be taken to ensure the tissues are apposed rather than everted, and the suture angle should be placed so that it passes just below the dermis. Mattress sutures can be modified to form a cross over or under the incision, i.e. a cruciate mattress suture (see Fig. 5.5).

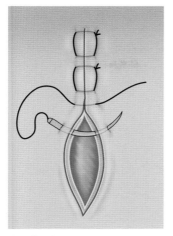

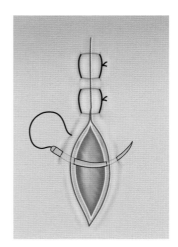

Figure 5.5   Cruciate mattress suture pattern

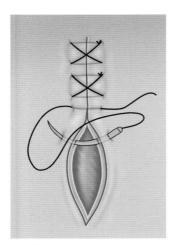

Figure 5.6   Vertical mattress suture pattern

Vertical mattress sutures (Fig. 5.6)

When placing a vertical mattress suture, the needle should be inserted approximately 8–10 mm from the wound edge on one side, passed across the incision line, and then exited at an equal distance on the opposite side of the incision. The position of the needle is then reversed and inserted through the skin on the same side exited, but approximately 4 mm from the skin edge across the incision line, and exits the skin again approximately 4 mm from the skin edge and the knot tied. This suture pattern is selected as it is stronger than horizontal mattress sutures, therefore making it particularly useful in areas where the skin is under tension. However, the placement of this suture pattern is time consuming, but it results in less tissue eversion of the skin margins than horizontal mattress sutures.

CONTINUOUS SUTURE PATTERNS

Simple continuous sutures (Fig. 5.7)

This suture pattern is composed of a series of simple interrupted sutures with a knot on either end; the suture is continuous between the knots. At the start of a simple continuous suture line, a simple interrupted suture is placed and knotted; however, only the end that is not attached to the needle is cut. The needle is then inserted through the skin perpendicular to the incision. To end a simple continuous suture line, the needle end of the suture is tied to the last loop of the suture that is outside the tissues. If an eyed needle is being used, then the needle is passed through the tissue, and the short end of the suture is grasped. A loop of suture is pulled through with the needle, and this loop is tied to the single end on the contralateral side.

Simple continuous sutures are frequently used in the closure of the linea alba and subcutaneous tissues. Care must be taken when placing this suture in areas where tightening of the suture may result in the formation of a purse string suture.

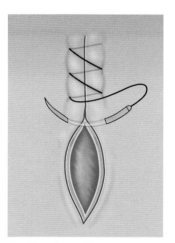 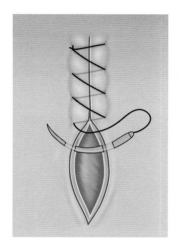

Figure 5.7 Simple continuous suture pattern

Ford interlocking suture (Fig. 5.8)

This pattern is a modification of the simple continuous suture pattern, where each time the suture passes through the tissues it is partly locked. To end this suture pattern, the needle is introduced in the opposite direction from that used previously, and the end is held on that side. The loop of suture material formed on that side is tied to the single end. Locked suture patterns have the advantage of being placed quickly and may result in better tissue apposition of tissues than simple interrupted suture patterns. This suture pattern does, however, use large amounts of suture material and may be difficult to remove.

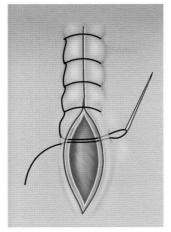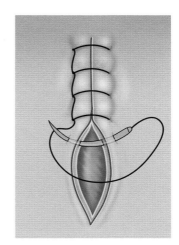

Figure 5.8   Ford interlocking suture pattern

Lembert pattern

The Lembert pattern is a variation of a vertical mattress suture pattern applied in a continuous pattern. This is an inverting suture pattern that is frequently used to close hollow viscera. The needle passes through the serosa and muscularis approximately 8–10 mm from the edge of the incision and exits near the wound edge on the same side. After passing over the incision, the needle penetrates approximately 3–4 mm from the wound edge and exits 8–10 mm away from the incision. This pattern is repeated along the length of the incision.

Connell and Cushing patterns

These suture patterns are frequently used to close hollow organs, as they result in tissue inversion and also result in a watertight seal. The Connell and Cushing patterns are similar, except that a Connell pattern enters into the lumen, with the Cushing pattern entering only the submucosal layer. The suture line is started with a simple interrupted or vertical mattress suture. The needle is advanced parallel to the incision and introduced into the serosa, passing through the muscular and mucosal surfaces. From the deep surface (the lumen with the Connell suture), the needle is advanced parallel along the incision and returned through the tissues to the serosal surface. Once outside the viscera, the needle and suture are passed across the incision and introduced at a point that corresponds to the exit point on the contralateral side. The suture is then repeated. The suture should cross the incision perpendicularly. When the suture is tightened, the incision inverts. A Parker-Kerr suture is a modification of the Cushing and Lembert patterns that has been advocated for closing the stump of hollow viscera. It is very rarely used as it results in excessive tissue inversion.

SUMMARY

It may seem slightly bewildering to have so many suture material choices available. Choosing the right material does not have to be such a daunting task.

- Consider the patient and any concurrent problems it may have as well as what type of tissues need to be closed, and how long these tissues will need support for.
- Think about suture size as well as suture material in your selection process.
- Thinking about the different materials by breaking them down into absorbable versus non-absorbable materials to serve your current need will often help make the choices simpler.

In the end, the choice may be narrowed down to several appropriate suture materials, and in such cases surgeons will often reach for the product with which they are familiar. Do not be pressured into making choices that make no sense; at the end of the day it is often the surgeon who will be losing sleep.

Table 5.1   Monofilament absorbable sutures

Brand name	Generic name	Action of absorption	Duration of tensile strength
PDS II™	Polydiaxanone	Hydrolysis	Loses 26% of its tensile strength by 14 days, 42% after 28 days and 86% after 56 days; absorption is complete after 182 days
Maxon™	Polyglyconate	Foreign body response	Loses 20% of its tensile strength after 7 days, 25% after 14 days, 35% after 21 days and 75% after 42 days; absorption is complete after 6 months
Biosyn™	Glycomer 631	Hydrolysis	Loses approximately 25% of USP minimum knot strength after 2 weeks and 60% after 3 weeks; absorption is complete at between 90 and 110 days
Monocryl™	Polyglecaprone 25	Hydrolysis	High initial tensile strength, rapid loss. 75% of initial tensile strength lost after 14 days; complete absorption after 4 months
Caprosyn™	Polyglytone 6211	Hydrolysis	Loses approximately 40–50% of USP minimum knot strength after 5 days and 70–80% after 10 days; absorption complete by 56 days
Surgical gut	Surgical gut	Foreign body response	Variable rate of absorption. Chromic gut longer, loses 50% tensile strength after 14 days, 100% after 28 days

Table 5.2   Braided absorbable sutures

Brand name	Generic name	Action of absorption	Duration of tensile strength
Vicryl™	Polyglactin 910	Hydrolysis	Loses 25% after 2 weeks, 50–60% after 3 weeks; complete absorption by 56 to 70 days
Polysorb™	Glycolide/lactide copolymer	Hydrolysis	Loses approximately 205 of USP minimum knot strength after 2 weeks and 70% after 3 weeks; absorption is complete by 56 to 70 days
Dexon™	Polyglycolic acid/polycaprolate	Hydrolysis	Loses 35% after 14 days, 65% within 21 days; complete absorption within 60 to 90 days

Further reading

Baines SJ 2004 Options for wound closure. VN Times, May 2004: 8-12

O'Sullivan J 1996 An introduction to suturing. Veterinary Nursing Journal 11(6): 180-189

Sissener T 2004 Suture materials and properties. UK Vet 9(6): 20-29

Chapter 6

Bandaging techniques and complications

Louise O'Dwyer

This chapter will describe and demonstrate the bandaging techniques with which veterinary nurses should be familiar and it will also describe techniques used for the bandaging of difficult wounds, e.g. skin grafts, where good bandaging techniques are essential for the immobilisation of the graft site. The chapter will also discuss the potential complications of poor bandaging techniques and how such situations can be avoided. Alternative techniques for the application of dressings will be described, e.g. the use of 'tie-over' bolus dressings.

BANDAGES AND DRESSINGS

The ongoing management of the wound to allow secondary closure, delayed primary closure or second intention healing involves protection of the wound surface by bandaging.

Bandaging aims to achieve the following:

■ Immobilisation of the wound surfaces, ensuring that the capillary buds and migrating epithelial cells are not disrupted and therefore maximising the rate of wound healing
■ Protection of the wound from trauma and contamination (including self-trauma and bacteria migrating through the dressing onto the wound)
■ Pain relief for the patient
■ First aid – bandaging of a wound may be a temporary first aid measure to protect the wound from further contamination and to aid haemostasis while a trauma patient is stabilised. The wound should be covered with a non-adherent dressing and an absorbent secondary layer. At this stage, ointments, antiseptics or wound powders may only serve to cause chemical damage and complicate debridement later on.

The most important layer of the dressing in terms of wound healing is the primary contact layer which should be chosen according to the condition of the wound. In the early stages, if the wound is still producing exudate and necrotic debris, debriding dressings are indicated. As the wound improves and granulation tissue is evident, a semi-occlusive, non-adherent dressing may be used which will allow exudate to be drawn away from the wound into the secondary layer of the bandage, while keeping the wound surface moist and protected. New tissue is not damaged on removal. Petroleum gauze products allow excess fluid through, but may allow slow epithelialisation. Smooth, non-adherent dressings, such as Melolin™ (Smith & Nephew), may be used as the exudate reduces.

Occlusive dressings are indicated once there is no infection and the wound is healing well. They keep the wound bed moist and warm and protect the new epithelium from abrasion. The hydrocolloids are a suspension of starch polymers in an adhesive matrix. They absorb fluid from the wound and form a moist gel. The edges of the dressing overlap with normal skin and form a seal, so that secondary dressing layers are not needed. This stimulates granulation tissue, allows rapid epithelialisation and also has some analgesic effect. Hydrocolloid dressings may prove expensive if dressing changes are frequent, but can be left in place for up to 5 days. These dressings will cause maceration of the tissue if the wound is exudative and they do not allow debridement. Furthermore, the adherence of the dressing at the wound edges may 'splint' the wound and prevent contraction. Intrasite™ gel (Smith & Nephew) is a hydrocolloid gel that may be used in a concave wound to allow the advantages of the moist environment but without being completely occlusive. The gel should be covered with a non-adherent dressing and a secondary absorbent layer.

Alginate dressings (e.g. Kaltostat™; BritCair™) also form a gel after absorbing wound exudate, and encourage epithelialisation in the same way. As they are not occlusive, they may be used as an alternative to the hydrocolloids if there is any doubt as to the state of the wound. Kaltostat™ may be useful for the transition from debriding dressings to hydrocolloids in the management of open wounds. The wound should be irrigated with sterile saline to remove the dressing.

All of these primary layer dressings are only as good as the bandage holding them in place. They must be changed regularly. It is important that the owner appreciates that if the bandage becomes wet it should be changed immediately.

Generally, bandages are composed of three basic component layers:

■ Primary (contact) layer
■ Secondary (intermediate) layer
■ Tertiary (outer) layer.

Primary layer

This involves the various dressings available for use as the contact layer; this has been discussed in Chapter 4.

Secondary (intermediate) layer

It is essential that all layers of a bandage are correctly and meticulously applied in order to avoid the common complications that can arise from inadequate, unskilled or incorrect application. The role of the secondary layer in wound management, in addition to providing support and comfort, is absorption. It acts as a 'trap' for exudative fluids from the wound; evaporation from this layer helps to prevent bacterial strikethrough. To aid its absorptive role this layer needs to have good capilliarity and should be thick enough (single or preferably multi-layered) to collect the fluid and pad the wound. The intermediate layer must be in close contact with the primary dressing but it should not be applied so tightly as to limit exudate absorption. Suitable materials are hospital quality absorbent cotton wool or synthetic materials.

Tertiary (outer) layer

The outer layer serves to hold all the other layers of the bandage in place. In a multi-layered bandage (e.g. modified Robert-Jones), intermediate layers of conforming gauze and absorbent material may be used prior to applying an outer covering such as an adhesive wrap or preferably a self-adhering dressing. It is important that the outer layer allows evaporation of fluid but minimises external fluid absorption. Plastic bags which may be placed over the distal dressing should only be left in situ for a minimal period to prevent excessive fluid retention, with the increased risk of bacterial strikethrough and tissue maceration.

TIE-OVER (BOLUS) DRESSING

Tie-over (bolus) dressings are a useful method of securing contact layers to all parts of the body, where conventional bandaging techniques are of limited value, e.g. the greater trochanter. The most common method of securing such a dressing is to use several loops of 3 metric (2/0) monofilament nylon sutures placed some 2 cm from the wound edge. Umbilical (nylon) tape is passed through these loops to secure the dressing; the tape is laced across the dressing through the skin sutures. Alternatively, long strands of suture material may be stapled 2 to 3 cm from the wound edges all around the edges of the wound; these sutures may then be tied over the dressing to hold it in place (Figs 6.1 & 6.2). The entire area should then be covered with an outer bandage, if possible.

Non-adherent dressing is applied to the wound, and cotton wool is then placed in the centre of the dressing. The edges of the dressing are then folded over and secured either with sutures or umbilical tape.

PRESSURE RELIEF BANDAGES

Pressure relief dressings are indicated for the prevention of decubital ulcer type lesions or treatment of superficial ulceration secondary to bandages or casts. Generally, doughnut-shaped and pipe insulation are employed to protect the area concerned by avoiding pressure over bony prominences (see Fig. 6.3). Care should be taken when using doughnut-shaped bandages, as they can in some instances be counterproductive as they produce a 'halo' compression of the skin around a bony prominence. This compression can occasionally be severe enough to compromise the circulation and therefore delay healing. Soft foam pad (pipe

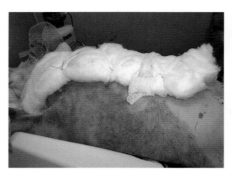

Figure 6.1   Placement of a tie-over dressing to allow the placement of a primary dressing layer and restrict the movement of the wound

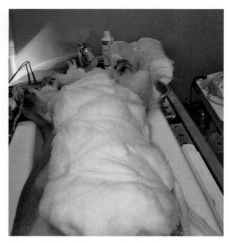

Figure 6.2   Placement of a tie-over dressing to allow the placement of a primary dressing layer and restrict the movement of the wound

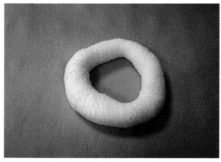

Figure 6.3   'Doughnut'-type pressure relief dressing

insulation) can be used parallel to the lesion so as not to encircle the wound so that circulation is not compromised.

ROBERT JONES BANDAGE

This bandage was named after a famous orthopedic surgeon, Sir Robert Jones (1858–1933); this type of bandage is used to support fractures of the limbs distal to the elbow or stifle. It is frequently used as a first aid measure or in combination with other methods of fixation. It is also highly useful in the prevention or reduction of oedema, and in restricting the movement of a limb.

Placement

Any wounds which are present on the limb should be suitably dressed. Two 2.5-cm adhesive, non-elastic strips, e.g. zinc oxide, are attached to the limb. These tape strips should be long enough to continue for 10–15 cm distal to the limb; these extended strips are later used to create the 'stirrups' which are used in order to prevent the bandage from falling down the limb (see Fig. 6.4A). The padding material is then applied evenly over the entire length of the limb, until the limb is approximately three times its original width. This padding layer should extend from the level of the toes and should extend proximally to include the joint proximal to the fracture (see Fig. 6.4B). The most widely used, and readily available material is cotton wool; this is cheap, and easy to compress and tear into suitable widths to allow for the natural angles and contours of the limb.

When placing such dressings on the hindlimbs, the leg should be slightly flexed before the padding layer is applied, so that the limb will not be dragged when the bandage is finished, as it is effectively longer than the opposite limb.

At least two layers of conforming or white open weave bandage should then be firmly applied over the cotton wool layer, working from the toes proximally (see Fig. 6.4C: conforming bandage, i.e. bandage which takes the shape of, or conforms well to the shape of the area in which the bandage is being applied). The bandage should be unrolled in short sections, always keeping the flat surface towards the limb; with each turn the bandage should overlap the previous turn by one half to two-thirds. The aim of this is to achieve an even, firm compression over the entire surface of the bandage. Any irregularities in the first layer of the bandage layer may be flattened by the second layer of bandage. The tape 'stirrups' are then folded back and stuck down on the bandage; these tape 'stirrups' will assist in preventing the dressing from slipping down (see Fig. 6.4D). If there is any excess cotton wool around the toes then this should be carefully removed and finally a protective layer of either adhesive elastic (Elastoplast™, Smith & Nephew) or cohesive bandage (e.g. Vetrap™, 3M Animalcare Products) should then be applied (see Fig. 6.4E and F). Ideally, it is said that the finished bandage should be resonant when flicked and sound like a 'ripe watermelon'. The central two toes should just protrude so they can easily be checked for their colour and temperature. Leaving the toes exposed also helps to encourage the patient to use the limb and allows for some weightbearing by the limb.

An alternative method of applying a Robert Jones type bandage is to alternate several layers of cotton wool and bandage. Such dressings are frequently applied in various thicknesses; thicker if external support is required for a fracture or lighter as a light support, to control swelling or to hold in place dressings which may be placed higher up the limb. Such modified support dressings may also include splints, which may be incorporated in between layers of padding material in order to prevent areas of pressure or rubbing, which may occur if the splint was placed beneath the padding layers. Sufficient padding should also be placed at the proximal and distal ends of the splint to prevent trauma to the patient's skin.

Such dressings should be checked approximately 2 hours after application to ensure that the toes are not swollen. The temperature and sensation of the digits can also be assessed. If the toes do begin to swell, then the distal end of the bandage should be loosened slightly or a pressure bandage applied to the foot for 12 to 24 hours. The bandage must be kept clean and dry. The dressing should be checked regularly and may be left in place for 7–14 days.

Care should be taken that such dressings are kept dry, as the cotton wool will act as a 'wick' on contact with moisture. The owner should be made aware of this and the bottom of the dressing should be covered with a plastic bag, old drip bag or specifically made 'bootee' whenever the animal goes outside. It should be ensured that this covering is removed once the animal returns to a dry environment, as long-term covering of the bandage with plastic would result in major skin complications.

HEAD AND EAR DRESSING

The majority of head and ear bandages are placed to protect an ear that may be haemorrhaging due to trauma or post-surgery. Similar bandages may be modified to cover the patient's eye following surgery or trauma.

Placement

The ear which is to be dressed should be reflected upwards over the patient's head (Fig. 6.5A). Any wounds which are present on the patient's ear/head should be covered with a suitable sterile dressing. A pad of cotton wool should be placed on top of the patient's head, with the ear then being reflected back onto the cotton wool pad; a further cotton wool pad should then be placed on top of the ear (Fig. 6.5B). It may also be useful to place a further cotton wool pad

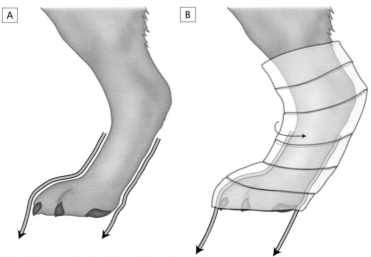

Figure 6.4   Placement of a Robert Jones bandage

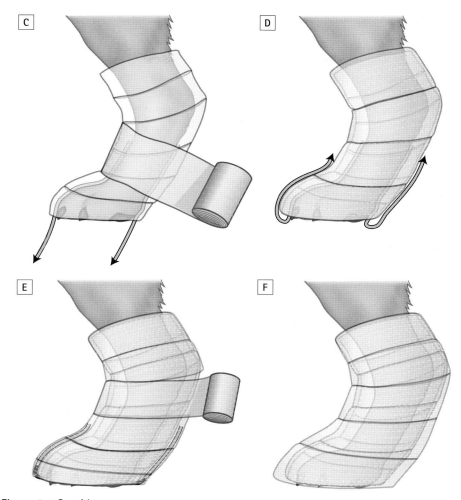

Figure 6.4 Cont'd

beneath the patient's throat, to prevent pressure from the conforming bandage and tertiary layer. A conforming bandage should then be used to secure the bandage in place. The bandage layer should start on top of the head, passing under the chin, in a figure-of-eight pattern. The patient's free ear should be used as an anchor, with the bandage passing around the free ear and over the head. It may require several layers of conforming bandage in order to secure the padding. A final tertiary layer of adhesive or conforming bandage should be placed in order to secure the dressing. If adhesive bandage is used then it may be useful to stick some of this bandage to the patient's hair in order to prevent the entire bandage from slipping forwards or backwards. A note should always be made on the bandage to show the position of the ear inside the bandage, to prevent laceration or even amputation of the pinna upon removal (Fig. 6.5C).

Whenever applying a head/ear bandage it is vitally important to ensure that the patient can still open its mouth and that respiration has not been impaired by the bandage being applied too tightly. It is particularly important that the adhesive layer is unwound prior to application; this is even more important if cohesive bandage is used, as if this bandage is applied under any tension, it can quickly become very tight, especially if more than a couple of layers are applied. If there is any cause for concern then the dressing should be removed and reapplied. Special care must be taken if the bandage is applied while the patient is anaesthetised, with an endotracheal tube in place, as problems may only be detected once this is removed. A correctly applied head bandage should allow the insertion of fingers between the bandage and the chin to allow room for neck flexion without obstructing the airway. If the bandage is too tight then an incision can be made partway across the bandage, under the chin.

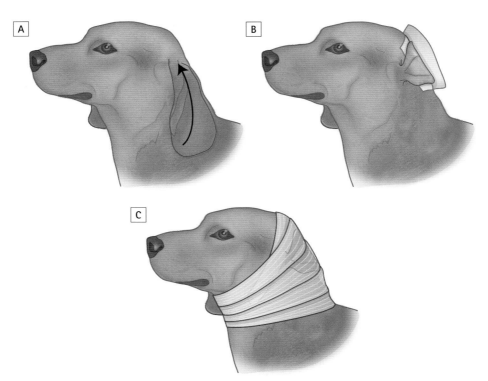

Figure 6.5   Head and ear dressings

If the patient is very persistent in its attempts to remove the dressing, it may be useful to extend the tertiary layer to include the cranial aspect of the chest, to prevent the removal of the dressing by anchoring it more securely around the shoulders, in a figure-of-eight pattern (like a chest bandage).

TAIL BANDAGE

This type of bandage is commonly applied following trauma to the tail tip, or postoperatively following amputation of the tail tip.

These bandages are commonly difficult to keep in position and can be very frustrating to place, especially if the patient wags its tail immediately following placement, and removes the dressing.

Placement

A suitable sterile dressing should be applied to any wounds (Fig. 6.6A). Many nursing texts advise the application of a layer of conforming bandage, covered with a layer of adhesive bandage, but the layer of conforming bandage commonly results in slippage of the bandage, so the proximal end of the adhesive bandage should incorporate the patient's coat in order to anchor the dressing (Fig. 6.6B). Other techniques for tail dressings include the placement of a syringe case of a 10- or 20-ml syringe barrel, with the tip removed, which may then be used to cover the tail tip and can be anchored to the tail using adhesive bandage (Fig. 6.6C), or pipe insulating material may be used to cover the tail, which again can be secured in place with adhesive bandage. This latter technique is useful as the pipe insulator is lightweight, therefore making it easier to secure the dressing in place.

FOOT BANDAGE

This is a commonly used dressing applied in an emergency to control haemorrhage and postoperatively to protect wounds and control swelling.

Placement

Cotton wool or other padding material should be placed between the patient's toes and beneath the dew claw. This padding helps to prevent pressure sores which may arise as a result of sweat from the glands in the foot and friction between the toes. It must be ensured that the pieces of padding are not too thick as this will make the overall dressing uncomfortable; at the same time strips must not be too thin.

Any wounds which may be present should be covered with a suitable dressing, then a padding layer should be applied over the whole of the carpus/tarsus; in foot bandages it is useful to extend the dressing as far proximally as the next joint, i.e. the carpal joint in the forelimb and hock joint in the hindlimb. This technique has the advantage of preventing the dressing from slipping down; however, care must be taken, particularly in the hindlimb, to prevent pressure points over the

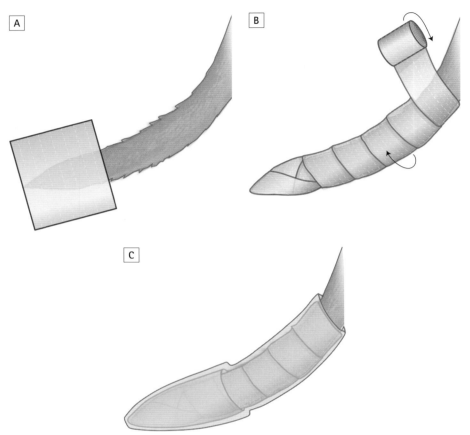

Figure 6.6 Placement of a tail bandage

hock which may result in ischaemic areas. The padding layer can be either cotton wool or a synthetic padding material, e.g. Soffban™ or Cellona™. It should be ensured that the padding layer is applied evenly. A layer of conforming bandage should then be used to secure the padding layer; this is the most suitable bandage for the secondary layer as it conforms well to the patient's limb and is generally easier to apply than other bandages, e.g. white open weave. A final layer should be added, using a cohesive bandage, e.g. Vetrap™ (3M Animalcare) or adhesive bandage, e.g. Elastoplast™ (Smith & Nephew). If adhesive bandage is used then it is useful to apply two shorter strips in a cranial to caudal, and then a lateral to medial direction; this will be useful to cover and protect the bottom of the bandage (see Fig. 6.7A–C). The remainder of the adhesive bandage can then be unwound around the remainder of the foot, with the bandage being applied distally, working upwards around the limb. It is wise to unwrap both cohesive and adhesive dressings partially in order to prevent the bandage being applied too tightly.

If this bandage is being applied to control haemorrhage, the bandage can be observed to detect bleeding of the limb through the outer layers of the bandage. If this situation arises, then a further layer of padding material may be applied, covered with layers of conforming bandage and then another tertiary layer, again with the bandage being observed for further bleeding.

THORAX AND ABDOMINAL BANDAGES

Such dressings are often placed to cover wounds, surgical incisions, drains or as pressure bandages in cases of suspected abdominal bleeding. These bandages need to be applied firmly, but at the same time ensuring there is no constriction of the chest or abdomen. When an abdominal pressure bandage is placed with the aim of controlling haemorrhage, the layers of the bandage should be applied firmly. It may be useful when removing such a bandage to do this very slowly,

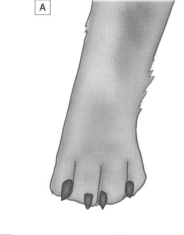

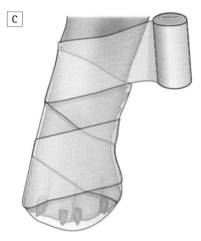

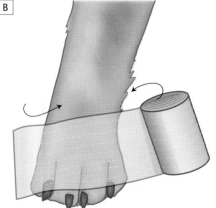

Figure 6.7   Placement of a foot bandage

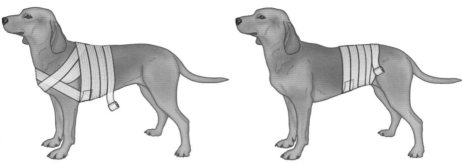

Figure 6.8   Placement of a thoracic bandage

Figure 6.9   Placement of an abdominal bandage

starting at the cranial end and making a 1-inch incision into the bandage every hour until the dressing is removed; this is generally done when there is a strong suspicion of abdominal bleeding (see Figs 6.8 and 6.9).

Placement

If a wound is present on the chest or abdomen then this should be covered with a suitable dressing, or if a discharging drain is present then suitable absorbent material should be used in order to absorb any exudate, e.g. sterile laparotomy swab. Several layers of padding material should then be applied; this padding layer should overlap by approximately half to one-third; this should then be secured in place with a layer of conforming bandage, and then a tertiary layer of cohesive or adhesive bandage. The dressing can be prevented from slipping backwards or forwards by wrapping the intermediate and tertiary layers between the legs and over the shoulders or hips in a crisscross fashion.

STOCKINETTE

One type of dressing which is incredibly useful and versatile in practice is stockinette, Surgifix™. This dressing is available in several sizes but only two sizes need to be kept in stock to dress any animal from a kitten to a St Bernard. It is most useful for patients with thoracostomy tubes in situ, as it allows easy access to the drain but keeps all attachments associated with the drain in place, hopefully preventing accidental removal of the drain. I have also used this dressing incorporated into chest/body bandages where regular dressings may slip, or where wound dressings require to be retained in place before further dressing layers can be applied.

Further reading

Williams JM 1999 Open wound management. BSAVA manual of canine and feline wound management and reconstruction, p 41-46

Chapter 7

Surgical drains

Louise O'Dwyer

This chapter will review and discuss the type of drains available, the indications for their use and potential complications. It will discuss the principles for placing drains, the choices available and the action of different types of drains. The chapter will discuss the techniques used in the placement of drains, how these drains should be managed from a nursing perspective, their removal and the complications which may arise as a result of incorrect placement, infection, patient interference and misuse.

SURGICAL DRAINS

A drain is a temporary surgical implant which provides and maintains an exit route to remove fluids or gases from a wound or body cavity. In veterinary use this may include air, blood, urine, pus, bile, chyle, exudate or serum.

Drains act by evacuating unwanted fluid from a wound and by preventing its accumulation. When correctly placed, drains will reduce the wound infection rate and encourage healing. However, by their very nature, drains are not inert, acting in effect as a foreign body; inappropriate use and care of drains may result in at best poor drainage or at worst death of the patient due to overwhelming infection and sepsis. Surgical drains have two main indications:

To eliminate the potential for dead space
To remove fluid accumulation from a wound.

ELIMINATION OF DEAD SPACE

Dead space can be defined as an abnormal space within a wound. Surgical procedures which involve the removal of large amounts of tissue and/or significant amounts of subcutaneous dissection result in wounds containing significant amounts of dead space. The elimination of tissue dead space promotes the early union of divided tissues and may be achieved by a combination of:

■ Surgical technique, i.e. the use of walking or tacking sutures
■ Pressure dressings
■ Surgical drains.

Drains should only be used if dead space cannot be closed and managed by surgical technique, e.g. walking sutures, or dressings.

The use of a surgical drain is suggested where:

- Fluid accumulation is likely to recur following simple mass removals, e.g. large lipomas
- Fluid cannot easily be removed, e.g. abscesses, bulla osteotomy, pyothorax
- Wounds cannot be completely debrided, and are thought to contain foreign material or necrotic debris
- Fluid will remain or be produced following surgery, e.g. skin flap
- Major wound contamination is inevitable, e.g. perineal surgery.

REMOVAL OF FLUID ACCUMULATION

If dead space is not correctly managed it will result in the accumulation of fluid within a wound. This fluid will compromise vascular supply and inhibit wound healing. In addition, an increase in wound infection rates may be seen as a result of:

- Reduction in the number of phagocytes reaching the wound
- The fluid present within the wound which will provide an ideal environment and medium for bacterial growth
- Opsonic activity by antibodies lost in fluid
- Local vascular supply possibly being affected due to a tamponade effect.

The presence of fluids in tissue may result in adverse tissue reactions or mechanical effects such as:

- The presence of a pleural effusion which compromises effective pulmonary ventilation
- Serous exudate beneath a skin pedicle flap which may prevent adherence to the underlying tissue
- Urine, bile or pancreatic secretions which have a direct irritant effect on the peritoneum leading to peritonitis.

MECHANISM OF ACTION

PASSIVE DRAINAGE

Passive drains act by providing a path of least resistance to the exterior of the patient. They function via:

- Overflow of fluid from the wound
- Gravity flow
- Capillary action.

The efficiency of a passive drain is determined by the size of its surface area. It is important that passive drains are placed dependently, therefore encouraging the movement of fluid away from the wound. The natural elasticity and movement of the patient's tissues will increase pressure within the wound and assist the movement of fluid along the drain. If necessary, additional pressure may be applied using an external dressing in order to encourage the capillary movement of fluid. The type of primary layer, e.g. use of sterile laparotomy swabs, may encourage capillary action. Passive drains should be avoided in some areas of the body, e.g. axillary and inguinal areas, as movement of the skin may result in air being drawn into the wound. Types of passive drains include Penrose, dental dam and corrugated drains.

Types of drains

In order to select the most appropriate drain for a particular patient's requirements, a good understanding of the drains available, their mode of action and efficiency for the removal of fluids or gas is necessary. Various factors need to be taken into consideration when selecting a surgical drain in order to ensure its success:

- Wound factors
- Patient factors
- Hospital environment
- Drainage systems
- Costs.

Types of drains available include:

- Surface acting drains, e.g. Penrose drains, corrugated drains, dental dams
- Tube drains
- Sump drains
- Sump-Penrose drains.

Surface acting drains

Penrose drains   This drain consists of a flattened, soft latex rubber tube and is available in a range of sizes from 1 cm diameter upwards and from 30 to 90 cm long (see Figs 7.1 and 7.2).

These drains allow some fluid to exit the wound via the lumen of the tube, but the majority of the fluid passes extraluminally, i.e. over the surface of the drain. Frequently, surgeons will add fenestrations to this type of drain in an effort to increase the rate of drainage; however, this practice is incorrect as it actually reduces the surface area and therefore its efficiency.

The placement of gauze tube within the lumen of a fenestrated Penrose drain will improve its capillary action through the wicking action of the material. This combination is known as the cigarette drain.

The Penrose drain is unsuited for suction drainage (e.g. thoracocentesis) as any negative pressure within the lumen will result in the collapse of the drain and therefore reduction in the drainage.

These drains are designed as passive drains and they function by removing fluid by gravity flow; as a result they must be positioned so they exit the wound

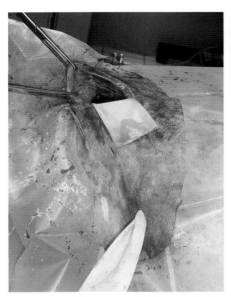

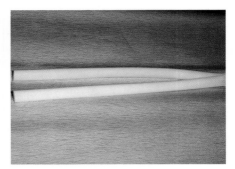

Figure 7.2   Penrose drain

Figure 7.1   Placement of a Penrose drain

in a dependent position, i.e. at the lowest point possible on the patient's body. The drain should be covered with an absorbable, sterile dressing, e.g. a sterile laparotomy swab, which will not only prevent ascending bacterial infection but will also improve the efficacy of the drain by increasing capillary action. Ideally, the sterile dressing should then be covered with further absorbent material, e.g. cotton wool, and then bandaged in place. This dressing will require frequent checking and changing, especially in the first few hours following drain placement as, if the wound has been lavaged with copious amounts of fluid, large volumes of exudate can be expected to be lost from the wound shortly after placement.

Corrugated drains   Corrugated drains consist of ribbed, malleable strips of PVC or rubber (see Fig. 7.3). They have no internal lumen and drainage occurs over their surface. As with all passive drains, their efficacy is determined by their large surface area and again they require dependent placement within the wound. Another type of corrugated drain is also available which does possess a central lumen, the Yeates tissue drain. This drain consists of a series of small tubes which are attached together to form a flat, corrugated sheet. This will allow drainage of fluids both over the external surface of the drain as well as via the lumen.

Tube drains

These are cylindrical drains which may be used as active or passive drains (see Fig. 7.4). They may be constructed from PVC, polyethylene, rubber, silicone or other plastics. They have at least one internal lumen and are available in a wide

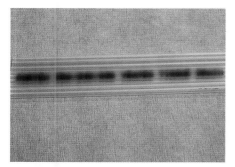

Figure 7.3   Corrugated drain

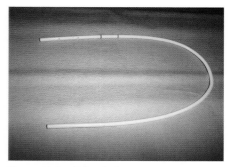

Figure 7.4   Tube drain

range of sizes from 3.5 to 40 French (1–13 mm internal diameter). These drains are much more rigid, in order to prevent the collapse of the drain when active suction is applied. As passive drains, they remove fluid intraluminally by gravity, with a small volume of fluid removed extraluminally by capillary action. When used as active drains they remove fluid only via the internal lumen. In order to prevent the collapse of the drain when suction is applied, they are manufactured from more rigid materials than the passive drains but unfortunately this means they are more likely to produce tissue irritation and reaction.

The section of the drain which lies within the wound is generally fenestrated in order to increase the efficiency of the fluid removal and to reduce the likelihood of obstruction by tissue or exudate. If a drain is selected which is non-fenestrated then fenestrations may be cut into the drain. These fenestrations should be oval in shape and should occupy no more than one-third of the circumference of the drain in order to prevent breakage or kinking.

Potential disadvantages of tube drains include occlusion of the lumen and collapse when suction is applied when used as an active drain. Red rubber tubes are found to be more irritant to the patient's tissues than other types of drains and materials; silicone rubber tubes are found to evoke a minimal tissue response.

Sump drains

These drains are in effect a tube drain with two or more lumina. They work by the larger lumen providing the channel for the movement of the egress from the wound, and the smaller lumen acting as a vent for the access and circulation of air into the wound. This venting action acts by reducing the likelihood of tube occlusion and increases the efficiency of drainage by displacing fluid from within the wound. The more lumina a drain possesses, the greater the efficacy of the drain. Sump drains are generally used for the removal of fluid from abdominal cavities (e.g. the peritoneal cavity) rather than the removal of fluid from wounds. When used in this situation they are more effective for the removal of fluid than Penrose or tube drains. The obvious main disadvantage is the opportunity for bacterial contamination of the wound via the ingress channel. To prevent this, the drain should be fitted with a bacterial filter. Foley catheters can be modified for use as a sump drain.

Sump–Penrose drains

This is a triple-lumen drain which is created by placing a double lumen sump drain inside a Penrose drain (see Fig. 7.5). On this occasion, the Penrose drain may be fenestrated, and gauze padding may be incorporated between the Penrose drain and the sump drain (similarly to the cigarette drain) in order to increase the capillary action of the drain and to reduce the tissue irritation and trauma of the more rigid sump drain. The Penrose drain is attached by encircling sutures at either end. The outer fenestrated Penrose drain allows fluid to exit whilst preventing tissue adherence to the sump drain. This design allows the drains to remain functional in tissues for long periods.

Modified Sump-Penrose drain

This contains another tube within the Penrose drain. These are more available commercially, or may be made by adding a rubber urethral catheter to the Penrose-Foley catheter previously outlined. The presence of three lumina also allows suction to be applied to one lumen, an irrigating fluid to be introduced via the second and air to enter via the third.

ACTIVE DRAINAGE

Active drains rely upon an external source of suction in order to remove fluid from within a wound; these drains are suitable for the removal of both fluid and air. The vacuum required for suction drains should just be sufficient to obliterate the tissue dead space; this is normally around 80 mmHg. If a greater pressure than this is exerted tissue damage may occur and/or obstruction and collapse of the drain is likely to occur.

Unlike passive drains, the sole exit for the drained material is via the central lumen of the drain, therefore all active drains must have a tubular construction.

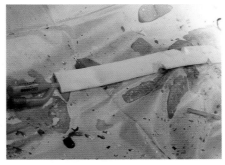

Figure 7.5   Creation of a modified sump drain using a Foley catheter inside a Penrose drain.

Active drains are particularly useful where:

- Large volumes of fluid or air are likely to require removal
- Dependent drainage of a wound is difficult to obtain
- Large amounts of movement are likely around the drainage site, e.g. axilla or inguinal wounds.

Suction may be applied to active drains either continuously at a low level (e.g. for the management of wounds) or intermittently (e.g. during thoracocentesis for a pyothorax). Continuous low suction allows an uninterrupted flow of fluid from a wound, therefore reducing the incidence of drain occlusion, the need for irrigation and the length of the drainage period. Continuous drainage systems allow wounds to be covered with dressings that will remain drier and therefore require less frequent dressing changes. In addition, the risk of bacterial contamination of the wound is reduced as ascending infection is less likely. One potential disadvantage of the use of continuous drainage is the risk of accidental disconnection, particularly in patients where thoracostomy drains have been placed.

A wide variety of suction systems are available for use with active drains, as described below.

Compressible plastic containers (e.g. Grenade™ continuous suction bulb, Global)

These systems are relatively cheap and simple to operate; they provide continuous and relatively uniform suction pressures. They work by being compressed, and therefore by the air being removed from the reservoir bulb, prior to connection to the drain (see Figs 7.6 and 7.7). They can be dressed into place for use in the ambulatory patient and may provide continuous suction for up to 24 hours (varying sizes are available depending upon the expected amount of fluid to be removed) under aseptic conditions before they require emptying.

Home-made devices

If none of the above systems are available in practice it is possible to construct suitable devices. This can be achieved by connecting a glass blood vacutainer to a butterfly needle (see Fig. 7.8). The extension tubing should be carefully fenestrated and the luer lock removed from the end of the tubing. The extension tubing is then implanted within the wound, as a tube drain, and secured to the skin using a purse string suture and Chinese finger trap suture. The needle is then pushed into the lid of the vacutainer and secured in place with tape. The entire vacutainer should then be wrapped in cotton wool in case of accidental breakage, and attached to the patient using a suitable dressing or bandage – Surgifix™ (3M, Arnolds) is particularly useful for such dressings. The vacutainer will require checking regularly and replacing as necessary; it is important to remember to kink the extension tubing before removing the needle from the vacutainer to prevent air being drawn into the wound.

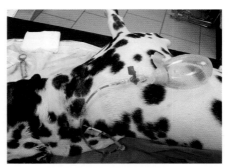

Figure 7.7   Grenade™ drain in place to allow active drainage of a seroma

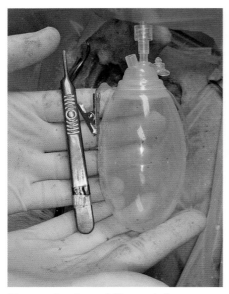

Figure 7.6   Grenade™ type drain

A similar device may be constructed from a 20–100 ml syringe, if a vacutainer is unavailable. The syringe is connected to an extension set, which should have the distal end removed and fenestrations created in the distal one-third of its length (see Fig. 7.9). The tubing should be placed within the wound prior to closure. Once closure is completed, the extension tubing should be connected to the syringe of choice, and the plunger withdrawn to create a vacuum. A large needle, e.g. 19 gauge, should be pushed through the plastic of the plunger so it sits just behind the barrel of the syringe, therefore retaining the vacuum within the syringe. The whole device then needs to be dressed in place with sufficient padding to prevent accidental trauma to the patient.

DRAIN PLACEMENT AND MANAGEMENT

General guidelines should be followed regarding the placement of drains and their management:

- The ideal drain should be made from soft, inert radio-opaque material which will induce minimal tissue reaction.
- When placing drains, they should not exit via the primary incision as this may interfere with the healing of the wound.
- The drain should never be placed near major neurovascular bundles or anastomotic sites, as this may result in the erosion of these structures.
- Contact between the suture line and the drain should be avoided.

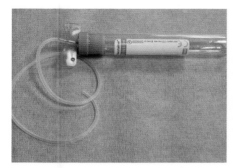

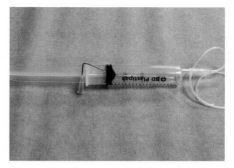

Figure 7.8   Home-made active suction drain using a blood vacutainer and butterfly needle

Figure 7.9   Home-made active suction drain using syringe and tubing

■ When placing sutures to close the wound, care needs to be taken to prevent incorporating the drain.

■ When using surface acting drains, the exit holes need to be large enough to allow adequate drainage but at the same time should not be so large as to risk the herniation of tissue from the wound.

■ The minimum number of exit holes should be used, which should be placed dependently if passive drains are used.

■ A large area of hair should be clipped from around the wound, particularly around the dependently placed exit hole of passive drains.

■ Barrier sprays, e.g. Cavilon™, or if unavailable, petroleum jelly, should be applied around the exit hole in order to prevent tissue excoriation; care needs to be taken to ensure the exit hole does not become occluded.

■ Strict aseptic techniques should be applied in the postoperative care and management of drains.

■ The protruding drain and the exit holes should be cleaned at least twice daily to ensure the exit hole does not become obstructed and impede drainage, and to reduce the risk of ascending infection.

■ A sterile dressing and a light bandage should be applied and changed as often as is required in order to maintain asepsis.

■ Suction devices should be changed or emptied as often as required in order to maintain suction.

SURGICAL TECHNIQUES

Placement of Penrose drains

Penrose drains are probably the most commonly used passive drains in small animal practice; they are commonly chosen for surgical or infected wounds. These drains should be anchored proximally within the wound using mono-filament absorbable suture material (see Fig. 7.10). A very small bite should be taken from the end of the wound; this is done so that when the drain is removed by tugging sharply, the drain will tear easily, without leaving a small piece of the latex drain within the wound, which would provoke a foreign body reaction, sinus tract formation and necessitate surgical exploration to allow removal. Another method of anchoring the drain within the wound is to place a suture of monofilament non-absorbable suture through the patient's skin, taking a bite of the suture and then exiting through the patient's skin again. This allows the removal of the drain by cutting the suture and again removing the drain using sharp traction. The drain should exit via a stab incision made separately away from the primary incision in a dependent position. Approximately 2–3 cm of the drain should be left protruding from the exit hole. This distal end of the drain should then be anchored to the skin using a single, monofilament suture. If a wound is large then it may be necessary to place more than one drain; again they should always be positioned and placed so the exit hole is positioned away from the primary wound, in a dependent position, to ensure adequate drainage (see Fig. 7.11).

Use of tube drains

One use of tube drains which is particularly useful is their placement following limb amputation. The fenestrated section of the drain is located within the remaining stump of the limb and is secured at the skin surface using a Chinese finger trap suture. This allows the drain to act as a passive drain, preventing the accumulation of fluids within the wound and removing dead space, but it also serves to provide

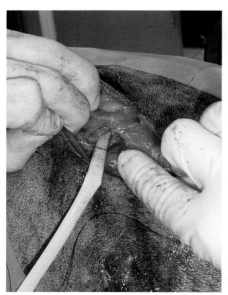

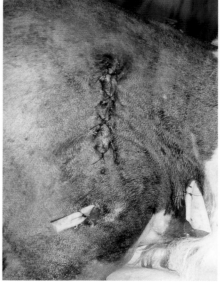

Figure 7.10   Penrose drain placement – the drain should be anchored within the wound at its highest point to encourage drainage from the wound

Figure 7.11   Final placement of the drain

a means of providing local regional analgesia to the surgical site with the instillation of local analgesic, e.g. bupivacaine, as the local anaesthetic exits the drain via the various fenestrations. This drain used in practice provides excellent analgesia to the patient, when combined with systemic analgesics, e.g. opioids and non-steroidal anti-inflammatory drugs, meaning a happier, more comfortable patient with improved recovery times and shorter hospitalisation times.

Using a tube drain in this way means that the drain cannot be left open-ended as a passive drain, but instead should have the end occluded (possibly with the use of an intermittent injection cap, which will allow the drain to be used intermittently as an active drain, and will also assist in the prevention of the introduction of infection each time the drain is used.

Tube drains may also be used as part of an active drainage system following mass removal or skin graft/flap surgery.

Drain removal

According to general guidelines, drains should be left in place until the drainage subsides. The drain should be inspected regularly and the amount of fluid in the reservoir of the dressing noted. This may be done by weighing the dressing prior to application, along with any additional padding material, e.g. cotton wool, making a note of this weight on the patient's records and then weighing these dressings upon removal at dressing change. All drains incite a foreign body reaction which results in the production of fluid. This means there will always be some fluid present at the exit port of the drain; this may be up to 50 ml per day in a large wound. Drains should be removed as soon as possible to reduce the possibility of wound contamination and the development of a sinus tract, which generally takes 3–5 days to form. The drain should be removed by cutting the skin suture and then quickly pulling the drain out of the wound whilst placing light pressure over the hole. A light dressing can then be placed over the exit wound, e.g. Primapore™, to prevent contamination. The wound can then be allowed to granulate. Thoracic drains should have a purse string suture pre-placed in the skin in order to close the skin round the wound quickly following removal. Some authorities recommend the instillation of local anaesthetic, e.g. lidocaine (lignocaine) or bupivacaine, 20–30 minutes prior to removal of thoracic drains; this is a particularly useful technique for less stoic patients.

COMPLICATIONS

It is important to realise that drains are not benign. If used incorrectly, the complications associated with drain placement may be more serious than the problem they were used to treat. Complications include:

- Wound infection
- Wound dehiscence
- Premature loss or retention of the drain
- Failure of drainage

- Pain and irritation
- Drain tract cellulitis.

Wound infection

The placement of a drain increases the risk of wound infection. The actual presence of a drain within a wound will result in the impairment of the local tissue resistance to bacterial infection because of the foreign body reaction, pressure ischaemia and tissue adhesion breakdown at drain removal. The exit hole increases the risk of bacteria gaining access to the wound. The infection rate increases directly in relation to the duration of drainage, and this infection rate increases further if passive drains are used compared with closed drainage systems.

Such complications can be minimised with adherence to strict aseptic techniques when placing and managing the drain. A large area surrounding the wound should be clipped, a barrier spray applied and sterile dressing used to cover the wound. The fewest number and smallest diameter of drains compatible with good drainage should be selected. The drains should be carefully placed in order to minimise movement of the drain, e.g. axillary regions, and should be left in place for the minimum length of time necessary.

Wound dehiscence

There is an increased risk of incisional dehiscence and herniation of tissues if drains are placed so they exit via the primary wound, or if large exit holes are made. Drains should be placed through a separate stab incision, which should be made as small as possible but at the same time still allow good drainage.

Premature loss or retention

Inadequate fixation of the drain may result in the drain accidentally falling out, or the patient removing the drain. In addition, if the drain remains in place for more than a few days, strong adhesions may form within the wound; if a large bite of the drain is taken or if the surgeon has fenestrated the drain, these factors may result in the breakage of the drain within the wound.

Records should always be made noting the type, number, size and length of drains placed. Efforts should always be made to ensure the drain has been securely placed and efforts should be taken to prevent patient interference, e.g. dressings and Elizabethan collars. Some drains, e.g. thoracostomy drains, have the additional advantage of having a radio-opaque marker present which will allow their detection should any portion of the drain be accidentally retained within the wound.

Failure of drainage

Inadequate drainage is usually the result of one of the following:

- Incorrect drain placement
- Use of incorrect (too small) tube diameter

- Loss of negative pressure within an active suction system, as a result of detachment of the drain from the suction unit or overfilling of the reservoir
- Obstruction of the drain with exudate, omentum, etc.
- Premature removal.

In the majority of cases the loss of negative pressure can be corrected by simply re-attaching another reservoir, or emptying the one already attached.

If a tube drain has become obstructed by tissue or exudate, it may be possible to remove such an obstruction by retropulsion, i.e. flushing the drain with a small volume of saline. However, care needs to be taken to prevent introducing contamination, so if this is necessary aseptic technique should be adhered to at all times. If the drain is present in contaminated or infected tissue, e.g. abscess, then the drainage of the wound will be necessary and such flushing would be indicated. The removal of an obstructed drain may be indicated and if continued drainage is required the placement of another drain will be necessary. If such problems are anticipated, the use of a fenestrated drain would reduce this complication.

Pain and irritation

The actual presence of a drain within a wound will evoke some irritation and pain, and may be responsible for postoperative pyrexia. This irritation and pain may be sufficient to cause the patient to remove the drain and mutilate the wound. For this reason suitable analgesia and protection of the drain should be provided.

Drain tract cellulitis

This is a problem frequently encountered with drain placement. Clinical signs include pain, reddening and swelling at the drain exit hole. The likelihood and severity of the inflammation increase the longer the drain is left in place, but generally resolve once the drain is removed. Strict aseptic techniques and careful nursing of drains should always be adhered to in order to prevent such problems, as well as the removal of the drain as soon as is possible.

Misuse and over-reliance

Reliance on drains should not be used to compensate for incorrect intraoperative or postoperative management. Drains are no substitute for proper haemostasis, gentle tissue handling and adequate debridement and lavage. Drains should not be used to compensate for closing a wound which would be better off left open.

- Drains exiting through the primary incision are associated with an increased incidence of wound dehiscence.
- The incidence of wound infection may be increased because of the risk of ascending infection.
- Obstruction of the drains may cause the retention of fluid or gas within tissue.

■ Drains which are manufactured from irritant materials, such as red rubber or PVC tubing which has been sterilised with ethylene oxide, are likely to cause local reactions leading to inflammation, ulceration and adhesions.

MINIMISING COMPLICATIONS

■ Strict asepsis should be observed during all handling and dressing of drains and their associated wounds. Wounds should be cleaned regularly each day and it may be advantageous to apply barrier sprays to prevent excoriation.

■ Drains should be left in situ for the minimum possible length of time so as to be effective. Always note the date on the patient's record when a drain is inserted.

■ Use drains manufactured from inert and soft material.

■ Ensure all drains contain a radio-opaque marker.

■ Drains should be measured on insertion so as to ensure the whole drain is removed.

■ Irrigation via a drain should be avoided because this may introduce contamination and increase the risk of asepsis.

■ Elizabethan collars as well as dressings over the drain will reduce patient interference.

Further reading

Baines SJ 1999 Surgical drains. In: Fowler D, Williams JM (eds) Manual of canine and feline wound management and reconstruction. British Small Animal Veterinary Association, Cheltenham, England, p 47-55

McHugh D, White R, Williams J 1992 Use of drains in small animal surgery. In Practice 14: 73-81

Chapter 8
Wound healing complications
Louise O'Dwyer

This chapter will discuss the potential complications which may occur in wound healing. The type of complication may take many different forms including post-operative haemorrhage, haematomas, seromas, oedema, wound dehiscence, infection, delayed/incomplete healing and the problems which arise as a result of wound contracture. This chapter will discuss the possible reasons why these problems may arise, the methods which may be used to treat them and the potential outcomes.

WOUND CONTAMINATION

It is estimated that 5% of all animals that undergo surgery develop infection despite all measures taken to minimise contamination and the use of prophylactic antibiotics.

All surgical wounds become contaminated with bacteria, but not all become infected. There is a critical level of contamination required before infection occurs; this is often quoted as approximately 105 organisms per gram of tissue or ml of fluid. However, there are various factors which are involved in determining whether a level of contamination within a wound will result in infection. These factors include: host resistance; characteristics of the contaminant organism and the interaction between the host and contaminating microorganism (i.e. local wound environment).

In order to assess potential risk of wound infection, patient evaluation should be carried out before any surgical procedure is considered. This evaluation will take into consideration the patient's physical condition, age, malnutrition, systemic disease, drug therapy and the presence of remote sites of infection.

The patient is generally the most common source of bacterial contamination via endogenous microbial flora. The skin and hair of the patient harbour significant numbers of endogenous and exogenous bacteria. The most common endogenous bacteria include *Staphylococcus, Micrococcus, Streptococcus, Actinobacter, Clostridium* and *Bacillus* species as well as some Gram negative bacilli and diptheroids. The range of exogenous bacteria present will depend upon the animal's environment and will therefore vary greatly between patients.

Wound healing is a very complicated process that takes place in four steps:

- Inflammation
- Epithelialisation
- Contraction
- Collagen formation.

These phases of wound healing are interrelated and may be influenced by various factors, including the local wound environment, i.e. wound dressing selection, and patient health, both of which can result in the delay and possible prevention of wound healing. There are also additional complications which may play a role in the healing process, such as the incorrect application of basic surgical principles, which will also affect wound healing. Technical considerations, including the use of sharp scissors, atraumatic tissue handling, minimal dissection, adequate debridement, achieving haemostasis and appropriate wound closure, all influence and promote successful wound repair. If these principles are not adhered to, then although the resulting complications may not be life threatening, they may, however, result in prolonged periods of veterinary care and patient discomfort and an increased cost to owners.

PERIOPERATIVE ANTIBIOTICS

The aim of perioperative antibiosis is to have effective levels of a suitable antibiotic present in the patient's tissues at the time of surgery and for approximately 3 hours post-surgery while the wound's fibrin seal forms. This means the antibiotic needs to be administered intravenously before induction of anaesthesia, and is designed to prevent the inevitable contaminants from establishing even a low level of infection. If the surgical time is prolonged then it may be necessary to repeat the dose of the antibiotic used. By using this protocol there should be no need for postoperative antibiotics for all clean and clean-contaminated procedures.

POSTOPERATIVE HAEMORRHAGE AND HAEMATOMAS

All surgical incisions will result in the disruption of the blood vessels; however the prevention of haemorrhage, as part of careful surgical technique, and therefore the prevention of subsequent haematoma formation, is more important than postoperative procedures to remove/limit haematomas. During surgery, the use of the correct size of ligatures or electrocautery can minimise haemorrhage. Minimising the amount of subcutaneous dissection will also assist in the prevention of the accumulation of blood within a space. If, during the recovery period, minimal incisional oozing is noticed, then this can be controlled with direct manual pressure for 10–15 minutes. However, moderate to severe bleeding will require the application of a pressure bandage or investigation and ligation of the bleeding vessels may be required. Once a haematoma has formed, its resolution may be accelerated by the application of a warm compress to the affected area for 10 minutes, three times daily. It will generally take approximately 7–10 days for the complete dissipation of the haematoma.

SEROMAS

The creation of 'dead space', as a result of either trauma or surgical dissection, may result in the accumulation of sterile fluids within that subcutaneous space; this is known as a seroma (see Fig. 8.1). The formation of seromas tends to be in areas which have redundant loosely attached skin, and are associated with excessive motion (shoulder, axilla and dorsum). Other than the presence of the fluid, seroma generally result in few other clinical signs. It is generally the owner rather than the patient for whom the presence of a seroma is more distressing. In some more specialised surgical procedures, e.g. skin reconstruction, the formation of a seroma may be detrimental to the adherence of the graft tissue to the wound bed. Seromas may also delay the healing times of affected tissues.

DIFFERENTIATING ABSCESSES FROM SEROMAS

It is important to be able to differentiate seromas from subcutaneous abscesses; however this may be done fairly simply. Seromas generally result in minimal clinical signs whereas abscesses result in intense local inflammation, including local skin reddening, oedema, heat, incision dehiscence, pyrexia and pain. However, the temptation to aspirate fluid to establish whether the swelling is due to seroma formation should be resisted, as this may result in the conversion of the pre-existing seroma into an abscess. If it is felt necessary to perform such a procedure then strict aseptic protocol should be followed, with the area being clipped and surgically prepared. Sterile gloves should be worn throughout the procedure and a sterile needle and syringe used in order to prevent the contamination and introduction of bacteria into the seroma. Any aspirated seromas should be monitored daily for further complications; however, it is highly likely that any seromas which have been aspirated will refill if suitable pressure is not applied to the site following aspiration, and owners should be advised accordingly.

PREVENTION

Seroma formation may be prevented with the gentle handling of tissues and careful elimination of dead space. If surgery will involve extensive soft tissue dissection and mobilisation, e.g. mastectomies or skin flap transfers, which would result in large amounts of dead space, subcutaneous sutures and active or passive drains or pressure dressing techniques may be used individually or in combination in order to prevent seroma formation.

Any seromas arising following surgery will generally not require any other treatment in terms of correction. Attempts at aspirating the contents of the seroma are generally pointless and may even result in contamination of the local environment. The placement of a drain may also result in further contamination and the seroma may even reform once the drain has been removed. Seromas will generally resolve without any intervention within approximately 2–4 weeks.

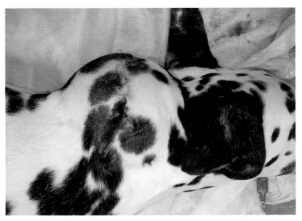

Figure 8.1 Development of a large seroma on the back of a patient's neck; active drainage was required (see Fig. 7.7)

OEDEMA

The wound healing process in the early stages is associated with inflammation. During this inflammatory process vascular and lymphatic obstruction and the presence of cell and plasma derived mediators will result in fluid exudate in the interstitial subcutaneous space, i.e. oedema. The extent of oedema formation tends to be greater in traumatic wounds than surgical wounds, but in surgically created wounds the surgical technique, extent of dissection and procedure performed may result in the presence of oedema in the first 3–4 days postoperatively.

Oedema may also be seen when large wounds present on the distal limbs are unsuitable for surgical closure and be allowed to heal via secondary intention. This process can often result in the impairment of lymphatic and venous drainage, and hence results in oedema formation. This is frequently the situation when the wound exceeds more than 50% of the circumference of the limb (see Fig. 8.2). The healing process results in contracture of the wound which in effect creates a tourniquet around the limb, resulting in swelling and oedema formation in the distal limb.

WOUND DEHISCENCE

The term dehiscence describes the breakdown of a surgically closed wound. This problem arises when, immediately following surgical closure of an incision, this incision becomes erythematous, oedematous or painful. A serosanguinous discharge may also result around the edge of the wound. It often takes 3–5 days postoperatively before the extent of the wound breakdown becomes more apparent, as areas of skin which have become necrotic and non-viable become increasingly obvious.

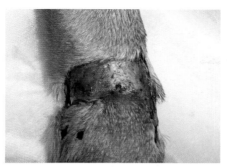

Figure 8.2   Wound extending around a limb which resulted in poor drainage of the distal limb

Wound dehiscence tends to arise due to incorrect surgical technique or methods of closure and poor wound bed preparation. The most common reason for the breakdown of traumatic wounds following closure is the incomplete debridement of all tissue which is contaminated or necrotic. All traumatically created wounds are considered as contaminated, if not dirty, wounds and therefore careful assessment and initial treatment of the wound should be made before its surgical closure.

CRUSH INJURIES

Crush injuries, such as those that arise as a result of dog bite injuries or vehicular degloving, as well as wounds which are heavily contaminated with organic material and debris, should not be closed primarily. Such injuries should be treated initially with 2–3 days of open wound management (see Ch. 2), in order to assess the full extent of the injury and the viability of the tissues and their suitability for inclusion in surgical closure. If attempts are made to close such wounds prior to this treatment it invariably leads to the breakdown of the wound due to underlying necrosis and infection.

LACERATIONS

Wounds which arise as a result of sharp lacerations are those more frequently treated in a surgical fashion by primary closure. This is not an incorrect surgical procedure to follow, however it is one which should only be followed once careful initial assessment and treatment of the wound has been performed (see Figs 8.3 and 8.4). The wound should be considered sterile throughout the procedure in order to prevent the introduction of infection into the wound. The wound should be carefully prepared for surgery as with any surgical procedure and care should be taken in its closure in order to prevent burying suture material deep within the wound as this could serve as a nidus or focus for infection. It may be appropriate to use a drain in the closure of the wound in order to eliminate dead space or this may be prevented with the use of appropriate pressure bandages if this is thought more suitable when closing traumatic wounds.

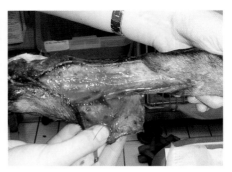

Figure 8.4 Laceration due to a patient stepping through a glass window pane

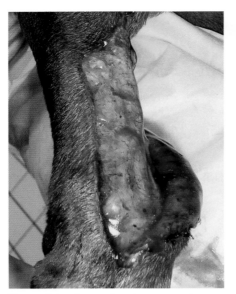

Figure 8.3 Laceration due to a patient stepping through a glass window pane

INCISIONAL WOUNDS

Incisional wounds may also break down, whether these are surgically created wounds or traumatically created wounds. This breakdown is frequently the result of incorrect surgical technique. If the wound involves the deep layers, e.g. abdominal muscle layers, and this wound layer breaks down then this may result in the herniation of the abdominal contents. This is one of the most serious situations in terms of wound breakdown (see Figs 8.5 and 8.6).

The prevention of this scenario can be achieved with careful surgical technique, appropriate selection of suture material type and size and careful and correct placement of knots, i.e. square knots rather than 'granny' or slip knots. The surgeon should also ensure that the correct number of throws are placed on the knots (see Ch. 5), and this is particularly important when continuous suture patterns are placed.

TREATMENT OF DEHISCENCE

When the situation arises where wound dehiscence has occurred, the situation should be assessed in order to identify any contributing factors which may have resulted in the condition. Where the wound has been created under traumatic conditions, the problem is frequently caused by any contaminants left in the wound or necrotic tissue which has not been debrided. This situation can be avoided by the careful assessment of the wound; see Chapter 2.

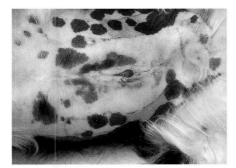

Figure 8.5   Breakdown of an incisional wound, allowing protrusion of subcutaneous fat layer

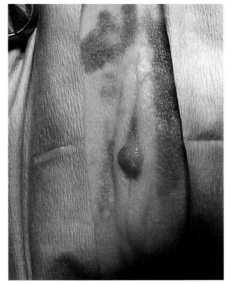

Figure 8.6   Breakdown of an incisional wound, allowing protrusion of subcutaneous fat layer

INFECTION

Any injury, either as a result of trauma or surgically created, which results in a break in the skin, will lead to bacterial contamination. In surveys, in approximately 5% of all surgical procedures in small animals and 2.5% of all clean surgeries, post-operative infection will occur (Vasseur 1988). In the majority of patients the host defence systems will phagocytose microbes and prevent infection. It is when bacterial levels exceed a critical level (>106 organisms per gram of tissue) that infection is highly likely to occur. Various factors can, however, affect the host's defence mechanisms and hence predispose the patient to infection; these factors can include local wound conditions and type of injury, bacteria contaminating the wound and the patient's status, including age, immune status (due to pre-existing disease) and concurrent illness/treatments.

Following injury, there is the infiltration of neutrophils and eventually macro-phages into the wound. These cells work together to destroy and phagocytose microbes present within the wound. If there are conditions present in the wound which prevent this action from occurring then this will result in infection within the wound.

The presence of wound infection will generally be evident 2–3 days post-operatively. Local signs of infection include heat, erythema, pain and oedema; the incision itself may have begun to open and there may also be the presence of a serosanguinous or purulent discharge. In addition to local signs, the patient may also demonstrate systemic signs including pyrexia, lethargy, depression and inappetance.

In order to appropriately treat postoperative infections, deep aspirates of the wound should be taken in order to isolate the bacterial species and perform antibiotic sensitivity testing so that the most appropriate antibiotic can be selected for administration. The aspiration should be collected as aseptically as possible, with the aseptic preparation of the patient, environment and operator.

Ideally, prevention of contamination of surgical wounds should be promoted, rather than the treatment of postoperative infections and subsequent complications. This can be achieved with the prevention of bacterial contamination within the operating suite, correct patient and surgeon preparation and careful and correct surgical techniques.

Such techniques may include those to reduce the presence of haematomas or seromas which would increase the risk of infection by providing ideal culture media for bacteria. Therefore the elimination of such conditions involves the placement of drains or suture material to reduce this dead space. However, there is a risk of infection associated with buried sutures, so this risk must be offset against the risk of infection as a result of haematoma or seroma formation (see Fig. 8.7). Studies have shown that more than one million staphylococcal bacteria are required to create infection when inoculated into normal subcutaneous tissue, whereas only 100 of the same bacteria in the presence of braided suture material would promote infection.

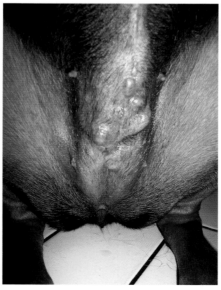

Figure 8.7   Suture material reaction

MRSA

Recently the incidence of Methicillin-resistant *Staphylococcus aureus* in hospitals has been rapidly increasing and the numbers of cases discovered in veterinary hospitals is also on the increase.

MRSA was discovered in the 1960s, with the strains of *Staphylococcus aureus* being particularly challenging for medical clinicians and microbiologists. MRSA is resistant to several other antimicrobial agents which include aminoglycosides, chloramphenicol, clindamycin, fluoroquinolones and macrolides.

The *Staphylococcus aureus* bacterium is commonly found in the noses of approximately 20–30% of the human population and is a normal commensal bacterium of skin flora. Of all *Staphylococcus aureus* found currently, only around 3% is MRSA.

The MRSA bacterium is usually confined to human hospitals, and is found particularly in vulnerable or debilitated patients. Such patients commonly include those in intensive care units, burns patients, surgical and orthopaedic wards. Patients who are particularly vulnerable include the elderly, diabetic patients and those with a depressed immune system. If the bacterium is in the nose or if it is associated with the lungs rather than the skin, then it may be passed around the hospital by droplet aerosol effect. This potential for transmission demonstrates the need for correct and thorough cleaning of the environment and the installation of correct ventilation systems in operating theatres.

The colonisation of healthcare personnel is asymptomatic and the main concern is transmission of the organism to these susceptible patients.

The prevention of MRSA when there is no illness or clinical evidence detected involves treatment using surface applied agents. This includes specific antibiotics such as mupirocin, applied inside the nose, as well as cleansing of the skin, and hair washing with disinfectants, such as chlorhexidine.

The main preventative measure within veterinary practice is meticulous handwashing and general hygiene, by all staff, before and after the handling of all patients. Disposable gloves should always be worn during the dressing and redressing of wounds.

CONCLUSION

Postoperative wound infections and wound dehiscence are beginning to be seen within veterinary practice. However, what is not known is whether this is a new problem or if MRSA has been present for some time within veterinary practice but it is only now that microbiologists are beginning to test for it, and hence are starting to isolate veterinary cases.

When wound infections present, a swab should be taken for culture and sensitivity in order to isolate the causal bacterium and hence enable the veterinary surgeon to know and prescribe antibiotics to which the bacterium is sensitive.

Staphylococcus aureus is commonly carried by asymptomatic humans, however the bacteria have serious pathogenic potential in susceptible individuals. The organism poses a particular problem due to its ability to develop and transfer antibacterial resistance through multiple mechanisms. This ability allows rapid adaptation to antibacterial exposure and the potential for multiple drug resistance. Resistance to penicillin was discovered 60 years ago and resistance to the next generation of anti-staphylococcal drugs was noted shortly after their introduction. Methicillin was first used in 1959 and the first resistant strain was reported in 1961. Methicillin resistant *Staphylococcus aureus* (MRSA) is not a new discovery but it is its increased prevalence in human hospitals in combination with the development of multiple antibiotic resistance that has resulted in increased mortality, morbidity and the cost of healthcare.

The recent public interest in MRSA has highlighted the importance of good personal and environmental hygiene in hospitals and this attitude is one which is of equal importance in the veterinary environment.

Staff should ensure that appropriate disinfectants and cleaning procedures are being followed; this should include the removal of organic matter prior to the use of disinfectants. Routine swabbing of theatres and associated furniture is also highly useful so that it can be ensured that the disinfectant being used is sensitive to the bacteria present in the surgical environment. This procedure is useful so that specific pathogens can be isolated and a suitable disinfectant selected. Screening of veterinary staff is also becoming increasingly popular, this procedure being carried out at many of the veterinary laboratories.

Ideally, practices should have standard protocols for cleaning to ensure this procedure is carried out correctly. These protocols should include areas which may normally be neglected during cleaning, such as the tops of cupboards, door handles, and insides of drawers. These are often areas which are frequently contaminated and handled and hence may act as a source of potential contamination.

Airborne contamination should also be considered; this can be minimised through wet misting of disinfectants, however this tends to settle very quickly and never tends to achieve an even distribution throughout the environment. Another step up from this is the use of an automatic disinfection unit, which distributes dry disinfectant into the air and throughout the environment.

One measure of which the public are highly aware in terms of attempting to reduce the incidence of MRSA in hospitals is the use of correct handwashing/disinfecting procedures and the use of hand gels or foams in between treatment of each patient. This same protocol should be applied to vets and nurses when dealing with animals.

Fomites should also be taken into consideration and disinfected in between patients; such items include the more obvious items such as feeding bowls, litter trays, bedding, etc. but items such as stethoscopes, pens, drip stands, etc. should also be considered in terms of their potential for infection.

When preparing patients for surgery it is not only the skin disinfectant which plays a role in reducing bacterial contamination, but it is also the method of preparation of the skin ready for surgery that should be taken into consideration.

If possible, sterile swabs should be used for the final scrub of the patient's skin once the patient is positioned in theatre; sterile containers should also be used as well as the correct concentration of disinfectant solution. The method the operator selects should also be considered, such as using the left hand to pass the clean swab to the right hand, therefore reducing the incidence of contamination in the remaining swabs and skin disinfectant solution. The operator should also wear sterile surgical gloves, particularly during this final scrub.

The surgeon should ensure the correct scrubbing up procedure is followed, whether this is a timed technique or brush count technique, and then correct gloving and gowning techniques should be followed.

Postoperatively, careful, aseptic wound care techniques should be used. Ideally, for at least the first 24 hours following surgery, the surgical site should be covered with an appropriate dressing while the wound forms a seal. If the dressing does become contaminated then this should be changed immediately before strike-through occurs, but again this should be done aseptically using sterile swabs and wearing sterile gloves.

The main aim of such aseptic and barrier nursing techniques is reducing the incidence of infection in wounds. Ultimately, if this is achieved then this means less need for administered antibiotics in order to control such infections. If antibiotics are only used when absolutely necessary then hopefully in the long term *Staphylococcus aureus* will not become resistant to other types of antibiotics. It should always be considered that domestic pets have the possibility of acting as a reservoir and may transmit MRSA to humans.

References and further reading

Ackerman N 2005 MRSA in your practice? Veterinary Nursing Journal 20(1): January 2005, 14-15

Duquette RA, Nuttall TJ 2004 Methicillin-resistant *Staphylococcus aureus* in dogs and cats: an emerging problem? Journal of Small Animal Practice 45, December 2004, 591-597

Remedios A 1999 Complications of wound healing. In: Fowler D, Williams JM (eds) Manual of canine and feline wound management and reconstruction, 1st edn. BSAVA, Cheltenham

Vasseur PB 1988 Surgical infection rates in dogs and cats. Veterinary Surgery 17: 60-64

Chapter 9
Wound closure techniques

Bruce Tatton

This chapter outlines the more routine wound closure techniques used in general practice. There will be a brief overview of some of the more advanced procedures that can be used in more difficult cases. These procedures are often carried out by specialist surgeons in referral centres. (For sources of more detailed information see References and Further Reading).

BASIC SURGICAL PRINCIPLES

As in all surgical procedures, basic rules of tissue handling should be observed. A useful summary of these are Halstead's principles:

- Atraumatic tissue handling. This includes the use of skin hooks and atraumatic tissue forceps such as Adson (see Fig. 9.1) or DeBakey forceps (see Fig. 9.2)
- Preservation of blood supply
- Surgical asepsis
- Anatomical approximation of tissues
- Obliteration of dead space
- Removal of necrotic tissue.

In cases of skin wound closure the following can also be added:

- Correct choice of suture material and suture pattern (see Ch. 5)
- Minimisation of skin tension
- Prevention of tissue desiccation during surgery
- Perioperative and postoperative nursing including analgesia, exercise restriction, prevention of patient wound interference, adequate nutrition and dressing management.

The physical condition of the patient affects wound healing. Larger wounds may be the result of significant trauma or disease and attention should be paid to the overall health status of the patient. Significant amounts of nursing may be needed and can make the difference between success and failure. Perioperative and intra-operative intravenous fluids may be needed, together with close anaesthetic monitoring.

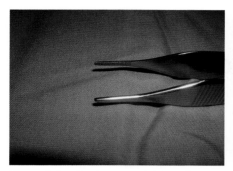

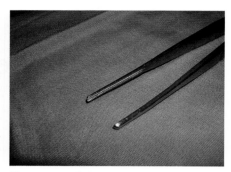

Figure 9.1 Finely serrated Adson tissue forceps

Figure 9.2 Debakey tissue forceps

CLOSURE OF SMALLER SKIN WOUNDS

UNDERMINING AND WALKING SUTURES

The wound edges should be in light apposition before skin sutures are placed, to minimise tension across the suture line. It may be necessary to undermine the skin edges to allow mobilisation of the skin. This should take place using blunt dissection beneath the panniculus muscle (where present) to preserve the blood supply to the mobilised skin via the subdermal plexus (see Ch. 3). In areas where this muscle is absent (e.g. the limbs) it is necessary to dissect under the fascia of the superficial musculature.

In wounds where larger areas of skin are undermined, and the skin is relatively mobile, walking sutures can be used. These are absorbable simple interrupted sutures placed underneath the skin at an angle between the hypodermis and the underlying fascia, in such a way that as the suture is tightened the skin is pulled to the centre of the wound (see Fig. 9.3). These also help to oppose dead space.

A balance has to be struck between the number of sutures necessary to draw the wound edges together and the fact that excess suture material can interfere with wound healing by acting as foreign material in the wound, and by interfering with the blood supply to the skin via the subdermal plexus. Some surgeons prefer not to use them if possible, as fixation of the skin to the underlying tissue may cause increased postoperative pain (Fowler 1999).

Intradermal sutures in either a simple continuous or simple interrupted pattern at the wound edges can be used to maintain apposition of the skin, reducing the tension on the skin sutures. During placement, occasional bites of the underlying tissue can be taken to help reduce dead space.

Simple interrupted skin sutures are the most versatile, allowing for staged removal of sutures if different parts of the wound heal at different rates. It should be possible to place the skin sutures relatively loosely to allow for postoperative wound swelling, without there being a gap between the wound edges. Too few skin sutures can result in inadequate wound closure; too many can interfere with

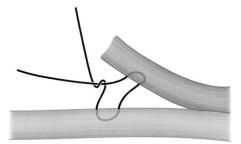

Figure 9.3   Placement of walking suture

healing as sutures act as a foreign material in the wound. An approximate guide for skin suturing with simple interrupted sutures is a tissue bite of 5 mm, with sutures 5 mm apart ('5 by 5').

Suture patterns regarded as being more resistant to tension (e.g. horizontal mattress) often seem to give poorer cosmetic results, and to be more uncomfortable for the patient. Rather than rely on these skin suture patterns to resist tension, it may be better to use techniques that reduce skin tension to a point that simple interrupted skin sutures can be used.

RELAXING INCISIONS

A single relaxing incision involves making an incision next to the wound that allows mobilisation of the skin between the two. The flap of skin created can be drawn over the original wound bed, allowing for primary closure. The surgical wound created is allowed to heal by second intention (see Fig. 9.4). This technique can be used to cover an awkward area such as a bony prominence. The relaxing incision should be placed to allow for easier healing.

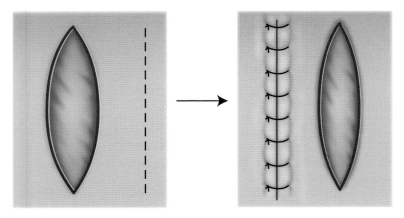

Figure 9.4   Single relaxing incision

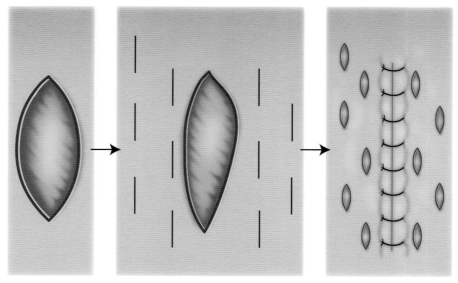

Figure 9.5   Multiple relaxing incisions

Multiple smaller (about 1 cm in length) relaxing incisions can be made, to allow for wound closure. The incisions should be placed in staggered rows to minimise damage to the skin blood supply. The multiple small incisions usually heal rapidly by second intention (see Fig. 9.5).

Other techniques for wound closure include circular wound closure techniques, V-, Y- and Z-plasties (see References and Further Reading).

CLOSURE OF LARGER SKIN WOUNDS

Closure of larger skin deficits requires more extensive mobilisation of skin into skin flaps. As with all wound closures the aim is to minimise tension across the wound line. Flaps which are too small will be under tension; this interferes with the blood supply to the wound, increasing risk of dehiscence.

Skin flaps are classified by their vascular supply into two groups: subdermal plexus flaps and axial pattern flaps.

SUBDERMAL PLEXUS FLAPS

Subdermal plexus flaps, as their name suggests, have a blood supply via the subdermal plexus which is maintained at their cutaneous attachment. They are raised adjacent to a wound and are useful in wounds located close to such structures as eyelids, anus or prepuce.

To try to avoid compromising the blood supply of the flap, subdermal plexus flaps should be at their widest at their base. There is no defined rule for the length of flap that can be raised relative to the base, but a length to width ratio of 2:1 is regarded as safe, with 3:1 as a maximum.

Subdermal plexus flaps should be undermined beneath the panniculus muscle (where present) to avoid damaging the subdermal plexus. In areas of the body where this is not present (e.g. the limbs), blunt dissection should include the superficial muscle fascia. Dead space underneath the flap can be closed with absorbable simple interrupted tacking sutures between the skin and subcutis. These should be limited in number to avoid damage to the subdermal plexus and some surgeons recommend avoiding their use altogether, preferring the use of active drains (see later).

Trimming the corners of the flaps to produce a slightly rounded profile, and using partially buried horizontal mattress skin sutures, helps to reduce necrosis of the corners.

Advancement or rotation of a flap can produce a fold of spare skin at its base known as a Bürow's triangle. Small Bürow's triangles can be left and will remodel, but larger triangles can increase dead space and interfere with wound healing. Techniques exist for their excision, and care should be taken to avoid interference with the base of the flap and its blood supply.

Subdermal plexus flaps can be divided into advancement flaps, rotation flaps, and transposition flaps.

Advancement flaps

A single pedicle advancement flap remains attached to the donor site by one of its margins. These can take the form of unilateral (Fig. 9.6) or bilateral flaps (Fig. 9.7) depending on the mobility of tissue on either side of the wound. Bipedicle advancement flaps maintain two cutaneous attachments. They are most often used on the limbs and the procedure should be planned so that this donor site can be left to heal by second intention (see Fig. 9.4). A single relaxing incision produces a bipedicle advancement flap.

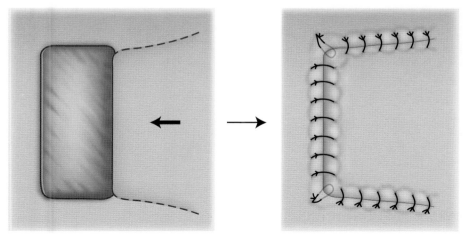

Figure 9.6   Unilateral single pedicle advancement flap (dotted lines indicate skin incisions)

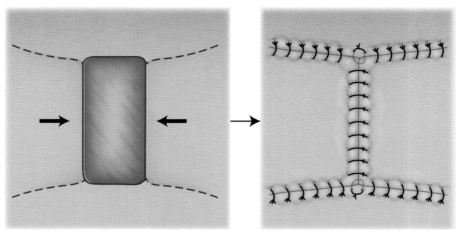

Figure 9.7   Bilateral single pedicle advancement flap (dotted lines indicate skin incisions)

Rotation flaps

Rotation flaps are elevated using a curved incision adjacent to the wound (see Fig. 9.8). The incision should be extended until the wound can be closed without excessive tension. The length of the incision usually needs to be about four times the width of the wound. They tend to be used in situations where the skin can only be mobilised on one side of the wound, e.g. around the anus.

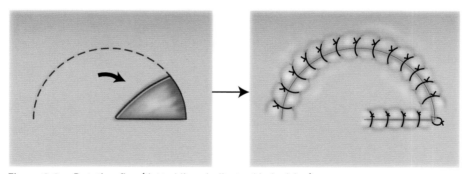

Figure 9.8   Rotation flap (dotted lines indicate skin incision)

Transposition flaps

Transposition flaps are developed at angles of up to 90° to the wound (see Fig. 9.9). They tend to be moved from the thoracic or abdominal skin to cover wounds affecting the proximal limbs.

AXIAL PATTERN FLAPS

Axial pattern flaps take advantage of the anatomy of the blood supply to the skin (see Ch. 3) by incorporating a direct cutaneous artery (DCA) and vein in their

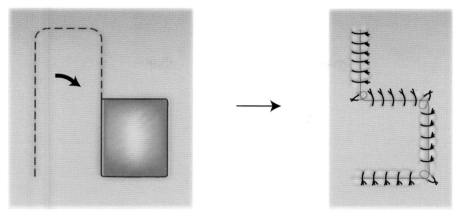

Figure 9.9   Transposition flap (dotted lines indicate skin incision)

design (Pavletic 1993). Clinically useful axial pattern flaps are based on the four or five larger vascular territories (or angiosomes) of certain direct cutaneous arteries (see Fig. 9.10). As a result of this more reliable blood supply, extensive

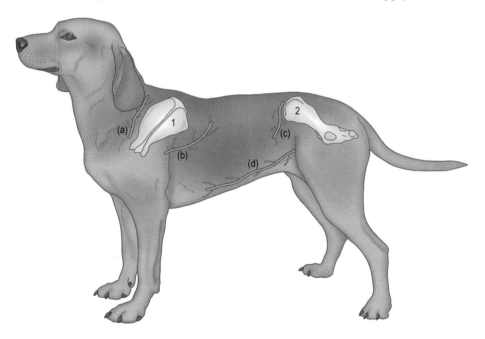

1	Scapula
2	Ileal wing
(a)	Superficial branch of omocervical artery
(b)	Thoracodorsal artery
(c)	Deep circumflex artery
(d)	Caudal superficial epigastric artery

Figure 9.10   Direct cutaneous arteries

areas of skin can be mobilised and elevated. The anatomical landmarks for the emergence of the DCAs into the subcutaneous tissues, and the orientation of the flaps that can be elevated have been described (Pavletic 1993).

Axial pattern flaps are used for substantial wounds with extensive skin deficits, and their use should be regarded as a major surgical procedure. Wide areas of skin need to be clipped and surgically prepared, and careful preoperative planning and marking of the boundaries of the skin flap to be raised is needed. Dissection should be deep to the panniculus muscle and great care is needed to avoid damaging the DCA. Unlike subdermal plexus flaps it is not necessary to maintain any cutaneous attachment for an axial pattern flap. This allows for a greater degree of rotation, and it is possible to rotate the vascular pedicle by up to 180°. If the vascular pedicle becomes kinked or placed under excessive tension, the blood supply to the whole flap can be compromised.

ACTIVE DRAINAGE OF SUBDERMAL AND AXIAL PATTERN SKIN FLAPS

The placement of large numbers of tacking sutures underneath the flap can potentially interfere with the blood supply of the flap. Depending on the location of the flap it may be possible to obliterate dead space with the use of dressings, but active drains can also be placed. These maintain constant suction in the wound, helping to appose the skin flap and the underlying tissues. Commercial drains are available (see Fig. 9.11). They can also be fashioned from a butterfly cannula and a syringe (Swaim & Henderson 1990). The needle is cut off and the tubing carefully fenestrated and the drain inserted under the flap and secured. The syringe is then attached and the plunger withdrawn to establish suction in the wound. Care needs to be taken to ensure that all fenestrated holes are beneath the flap, otherwise suction will not be established. The plunger is fixed in position by a suitably rigid tube or blunt-ended pin placed through a pre-drilled hole in the shaft of the plunger (see Fig. 9.12). As tissue fluid is drawn

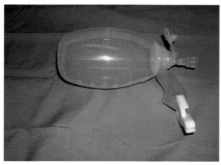

Figure 9.11   Commercial suction drain, Grenade™ continuous suction bulb (Global Veterinary Products)

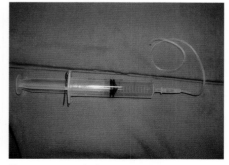

Figure 9.12   Syringe as an active suction drain with blunt-ended pin holding plunger in place

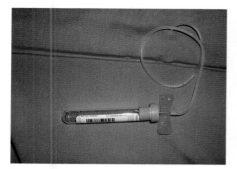

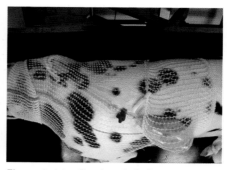

Figure 9.13   Vacuum blood collection tube used as an active suction drain

Figure 9.14   Suction drain incorporated into elasticated tubular net dressing

into the syringe, suction is lost, and the syringe has to be detached and emptied before being reapplied. Less squeamish owners can do this at home.

An alternative arrangement is to use a vacuum blood collection tube. In this case, the Luer lock is cut off the butterfly cannula and the needle inserted through the rubber cap of the tube (Fig. 9.13). The owner can be given a supply of these tubes and instructed to change them at regular intervals.

The suction drain has to be attached to the patient (Fig. 9.14) and is protected in a dressing, which usually takes the form of a body wrap. An outer layer of a tubular elasticated net dressing can be used to hold the dressing and suction drain in place.

References and further reading

Anderson D 1997 Practical approach to reconstruction of wounds in small animals, Part 1. In Practice 19(9): 463-471

Anderson D 1997 Practical approach to reconstruction of wounds in small animals, Part 2. In Practice 19(10): 537-545

Fowler JD 1999 Tension relieving techniques and local skin flaps. In: Fowler D, Williams JM (eds) Manual of canine and feline wound management and reconstruction. British Small Animal Veterinary Association Publications, Cheltenham, p 57-68

Fowler JD 2000 Skin flaps. In: Harari J (ed) Small animal surgery secrets, 1st edn. Hanley and Belfus, Philadelphia, USA, p 67-69

Harari J 2000 Control of infection. In: Harari J (ed) Small animal surgery secrets, 1st edn. Hanley and Belfus, Philadelphia, USA, p 6-11

Pavletic MM 1993 Pedicle grafts. In: Slatter DH (ed) Textbook of small animal surgery, 2nd edn. Vol. 1. WB Saunders, Philadelphia, USA. WB Saunders, p 295-340

Swaim SF, Henderson RA 1990 Wound management. In: Swaim SF, Henderson RA (eds) Small animal wound management. Lea and Febinger, London, p 32

Chapter 10
Skin grafts

Bruce Tatton

This chapter aims to provide a basic description of the skin grafts most commonly used in general practice. Only full thickness skin grafts will be described; split thickness skin graft procedures exist but are much less commonly used. The basic principles of surgical technique outlined in Chapter 9 also apply here.

A simple definition of a skin graft is a piece of skin that has been detached from its blood supply, and transferred to a wound bed where it subsequently develops a new blood supply. Skin grafts tend to be used most commonly on the distal parts of the limbs, where it is more difficult to close large wounds with local skin tension relieving techniques.

MAIN TYPES OF SKIN GRAFT

- Sheet grafts, which can be subdivided according to the degree of skin meshing as completely meshed, partially meshed or 'pie crusted' (Fig. 10.1). Unmeshed sheet grafts are rarely used.
- Strip grafts (Fig. 10.2A)
- Pinch/Punch grafts (Fig. 10.2B).

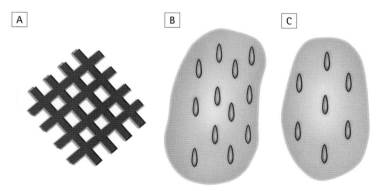

Figure 10.1   Complete (A), partial (B) and 'pie crusted' (C) meshed sheet grafts

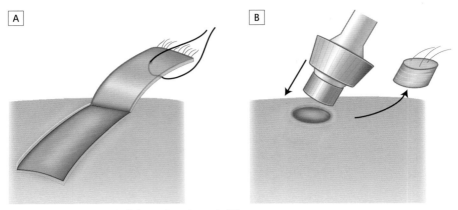

Figure 10.2   Strip graft (A) and Punch graft (B)

Factors to be considered for a successful graft include:

- Preparation of the wound bed, before and at the time of surgery
- Choice of donor site
- Harvesting and preparation of the skin graft(s)
- Attaching the skin graft(s)
- Postoperative management of the recipient and donor site.

The preparation and carrying out of a mesh graft will be described and the main differences with punch and strip grafting outlined.

MESHED SHEET GRAFTS

Preparation of the recipient site

Fresh surgical wounds can be grafted immediately after surgery (e.g. tumour removal) if the wound bed has a good blood supply. Often the graft is used to cover a more longstanding wound, and it is important that there is a bed of healthy active granulation tissue (which has a red roughened appearance and a more active blood supply). Chronic, inactive or infected granulation tissue does not provide a suitable site for a graft.

An inactive or infected wound bed should be treated as outlined in Chapter 4, to provide a healthy recipient site. Some 24–48 hours before surgery, using aseptic precautions, the wound should be gently scraped with a surgical blade to remove any non-viable tissue and coagulum. This also helps to reduce the bacterial load. The wound should then be dressed. A wet-to-dry dressing can be applied; some sources recommend the use of a 0.1% gentamicin sulphate ointment on sterile gauze. Secondary and tertiary bandage layers should be applied.

On the day of surgery the wound bed should be protected using sterile swabs soaked in Hartmann's solution, while the surrounding skin is widely clipped and cleaned using surgical preparation solutions. In established wounds it may be necessary to remove a rim of epithelium from around the wound bed. An incision is made around the wound at 90° to the tissue surface where the rim of epithelium meets haired skin. A second incision is then made parallel to the wound surface to undermine this rim of epithelium, which is then removed. Haemostasis is important; excessive haemorrhage can lead to separation of sutured wound edges, detachment of the graft, increased risk of infection, and delayed healing. Overuse of electrosurgery can result in devitalised tissue in the wound, which has to be removed by macrophages, delaying wound healing. The use of pressure or the clamping of bleeding vessels usually achieves adequate haemostasis with minimal tissue damage.

A piece of sterile paper or drape can be cut to the size and shape of the wound to provide a template. While the skin graft is removed from the donor site, the recipient site should be covered with swabs moistened with saline or Hartmann's solution, to prevent desiccation of the wound.

Choosing the donor site

The donor site is typically located on the lateral thoracic area. Here the skin is thin and elastic which allows for quicker revascularisation of the graft and there is hair, which allows for a more cosmetic end result. The skin in this area is relatively easy to mobilise and large wounds can be sutured closed. This site should be surgically prepared and draped, with a wide margin of hair removal.

Harvesting and preparing the skin graft

The template should be lined up on the donor site in such a way that when the graft is transferred, the hair growth at the recipient site is in the same direction as the surrounding skin. The template is drawn around using a sterile skin marker pen or a sterile cotton wool bud dipped in sterile stain such as methylthioninium chloride (Methylene Blue). A margin of 0.5–1 cm should be allowed around the template. The skin graft is removed using sharp dissection, dissecting superficial to the panniculus muscle. It is important to minimise traumatic damage to the graft tissue. The graft should be manipulated using skin hooks (bent 23–25 gauge hypodermic needles can be used, see Fig. 10.3), stay sutures or atraumatic tissue forceps (e.g. Adson or DeBakey forceps, see Figs 9.1 and 9.2).

The graft should be placed haired side down onto a piece of sterile cardboard or drape that allows the graft to be stretched by being fixed with sterile hypodermic needles or pins (see Fig. 10.4). The graft can also be stretched over the surgeon's fingers. Sharp dissection should be used to remove all the subcutaneous tissue until the dermal surface is exposed. This has a roughened appearance caused by the bulbs of the hair follicles. The graft can then be meshed. Although this can be done mechanically, in practice it is more often done using a No. 11 scalpel blade, the holes being about 1 cm long and in staggered rows about 0.5 cm apart. This produces a partially meshed graft.

Advantages of a meshed graft compared to a solid piece of skin include improved conformability to the wound bed, increased ability to expand the graft over a larger wound, and improved drainage of exudate from the wound surface through the mesh holes. Accumulation of tissue exudate from underneath non-meshed grafts can lead to detachment of the graft so the exudate has to be removed either by daily drainage via a hypodermic needle, or the placement of a

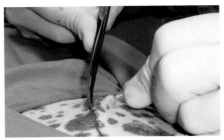

Figure 10.3   Manipulation of the graft using a hypodermic needle as a skin hook

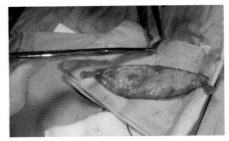

Figure 10.4   Graft placed epidermis down and pinned in place to allow removal of subdermal tissue

suction drain. One disadvantage of a meshed graft concerns its cosmetic appearance: the mesh holes remain hairless once healed.

Attaching the skin graft

The graft can then be positioned over the wound bed and sutured in place. Simple interrupted sutures of non-absorbable monofilament suture material are first placed around the wound edges, to hold the graft in place without excessive tension. Sutures can then be placed between the mesh holes into the wound tissue to fix the graft into position. These sutures help keep the graft immobile, allowing attachment and revascularisation (Fig. 10.5).

During graft preparation the donor site can be protected using sterile swabs moistened in Hartmann's solution. Routine donor site closure can be carried out after the graft has been transferred.

Postoperative management

The graft should be covered with a bandage consisting of a non-adherent primary layer, an absorbent secondary layer, and a protective tertiary layer. The dressing acts to keep the graft in contact with the wound bed, minimise graft movement,

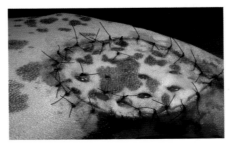

Figure 10.5   Graft sutured onto recipient wound bed

remove exudates from the graft and protect the graft from the environment. Splints can be added to the dressing, although care should be taken to ensure that there is not excessive pressure on the graft. It may be advisable to use precautions such as an Elizabethan collar to prevent patient interference with the dressing. The dressing should initially be changed after 48 hours, taking care not to disturb the graft. Subsequent dressing changes depend on the amount of exudate produced. This exudate should be serosanguinous. A purulent discharge may indicate a wound infection: swabs should be taken for bacterial culture and sensitivity, and aggressive antibiosis may be needed to try to save the graft. Accumulations of coagulum in the mesh holes can be carefully cleaned away using sterile cotton buds.

The graft should appear to be stable on the wound bed from an early stage. A little movement for the first 48 hours may be acceptable, but movement after this time prevents revascularisation. It is not unusual for the graft to have a pale or slightly bluish oedematous appearance for the first few days. If the graft is successful this begins to resolve and the graft takes on a more healthy appearance. Sometimes there can be a sloughing of the superficial epithelial layers. If the graft fails to 'take' it will start to change to a black or grey colour and fail to attach to the wound bed. The development of infection under the graft usually leads to graft failure (see Fig. 10.6).

After about 10 days it may be possible to remove the sutures holding the graft in place. This can be staggered over several days if there is any delay in healing. Devices such as Elizabethan collars should be kept in place for as long as needed to prevent self-trauma. Limited exercise and the use of emollient creams can help to reduce excessive fibrous tissue formation. It takes about 3 weeks for hair regrowth to begin and up to 6 weeks for the graft to regain the resilience of normal skin.

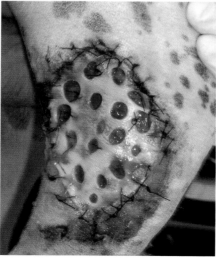

Figure 10.6   Failure of graft 'take'

STRIP GRAFTS

Strip grafting is less commonly used, and tends to be limited to wounds that are parallel to the long axis of the limb. There needs to be a bed of granulation tissue at the recipient site so that grooves can be cut into it to allow placement of the skin strips. These grooves should be about 5 mm wide and about 5 mm apart. The grafts are initially cut from the donor site leaving one shorter end attached. This allows the graft to be held under tension, facilitating the removal of sub-cutaneous tissue (see Fig. 10.2A). The grafts are then sutured into the grooves in the recipient bed using monofilament non-absorbable sutures placed at each end, and at intervals down the side of the strip. As they heal, the grafts revascularise and attach to the wound bed. The gap between the skin strips is covered by epithelium which grows from the graft edges.

PINCH/PUNCH GRAFTS

The grafts are usually prepared from the donor site in one of two ways. Either the skin is tented using a suture needle and the tip of the skin tent cut off using a scalpel (a 'pinch') or a Keyes biopsy punch is used to cut a 'punch' of skin. The biopsy punch can be angled slightly with the direction of hair growth, to try to include as many intact follicles as possible (see Fig. 10.2B).

At the recipient site, a scalpel blade is used to make a series of small pockets in the granulation tissue. The graft is then placed into the pocket. Alternatively, a biopsy punch of a slightly smaller diameter than that used to take the skin punch can be used to create a hole in the granulation tissue. Once bleeding has stopped, the skin plug is placed into the hole. Ideally the skin plug should sit just below the wound surface. Areas between the grafts heal by epithelium spreading from the graft edges.

Punch and strip grafts tend to heal quickly but the end result is not as cosmetic or durable as mesh grafts or skin flaps, due to the area of the wound bed that ends up covered in non-haired epithelium. Postoperative management for these two types of grafts is similar to meshed grafts although dressings tend not to be changed as often (perhaps every 3 to 5 days) to try to limit disruption of the grafts.

References and further reading

Anderson D 1997 Practical approach to reconstruction of wounds in small animal practice, Part 1. In Practice 19(9): 463-471

Anderson D 1997 Practical approach to reconstruction of wounds in small animal practice, Part 2. In Practice 19(10): 537-545

Swaim SF 2000 Skin grafts. In: Harari J (ed) Small animal surgery secrets, 1st edn. Hanley and Belfus, Philadelphia, USA, p 62-66

White RAS 1999 Skin grafting. In: Fowler D, Williams JM (eds) Manual of canine and feline wound management and reconstruction. BSAVA Publications, Cheltenham, p 83-94

Index

Note: Page numbers in **bold** refer to figures.